BASAL GANGLIA – AN INTEGRATIVE VIEW

Edited by **Fernando A. Barrios** and **Clemens Bauer**

Basal Ganglia – An Integrative View
http://dx.doi.org/10.5772/2976
Edited by Fernando A. Barrios and Clemens Bauer

Contributors

Gerry Leisman, Robert Melillo, Frederick R. Carrick, Clivel G. Charlton, M.O. Welcome, V.A. Pereverzev, Clemens C.C. Bauer, Erick H. Pasaye, Juan I. Romero-Romo, Fernando A. Barrios, Masahiko Takada, Eiji Hoshi, Yosuke Saga, Ken-ichi Inoue, Shigehiro Miyachi, Nobuhiko Hatanaka, Masahiko Inase, Atsushi Nambu

Published by InTech

Janeza Trdine 9, 51000 Rijeka, Croatia

Publishing Process Manager Dragana Manestar
Technical Editor InTech Prepress, Novi Sad
Cover InTech Design team

Edition 2014

Additional hard copies can be obtained from orders@intechopen.com

Basal Ganglia – An Integrative View, Edited by Fernando A. Barrios and Clemens Bauer
p. cm.
ISBN 978-953-51-0918-1

For EU product safety concerns:
IN TECH d.o.o., Prolaz Marije Krucifikse Kozulić 3, 51000 Rijeka, Croatia, info@intechopen.com or visit our website at intechopen.com.

Meet the editor

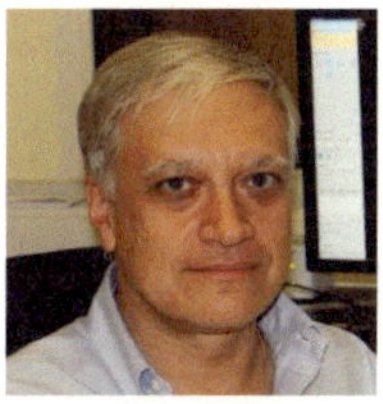

Fernando Alejandro Barrios was born in Mexico City in 1960, he attended the Science School of the National Autonomous University of Mexico (UNAM) where he was granted the Bachelor in Sciences studying Physics, in 1984. In 1986 he obtained the Master Degree in Sciences (Physics), at Ohio University, in 1990 he obtained his Ph.D. in Theoretical Physics at University of Cincinnati. After graduation he worked as posdoc with a Fogarty Fellowship at NIMH in functional brain mapping. At present time he is associate professor at the Neurobiology Institute, UNAM, and head of the Functional Brain Mapping Lab and member of the National System of Researchers, Mexico.

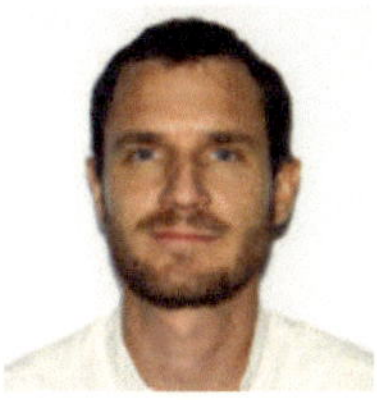

Clemens Christian Chimalpopoca Bauer was born in Querétaro Mexico in 1974. He obtained his M.D. from the Universidad Autonóma de Guadalajara. After some years as a General Practitioner he did a Master in Cognitive Science at the Universität Osnabrück, Germany. Currently he is a Docotorate Candidate in Biomedical Sciences at the Instituto de Neurobiología, Universidad Nacional Autónoma de México. Clemens Bauer has mayor interest in understanding the neurobiological correlates of self-consciousness. His studies include neurophenomenologic, behavioral and functional Magnetic Resonance (fMRI) imaging techniques with which he combines to approach this elusive field.

Contents

Preface

The study of the function of the Basal Ganglia is a subject of increasing prominence, not only among neuroscientists, neurologists, psychiatrists and cognitive-scientists but also for clinical ergonomists, rehabilitation, internal medicine and public health physicians. This work represents an attempt to bring together diverse scientists who are interested in a common subject, the Basal Ganglia, nevertheless are situated in different contexts in the scientific landscape. Basal Ganglia research in the last decade has been singled out with compelling findings, resulting in new ideas of related functional networks with other brain structures and internal functions that were not considered before. Many of these findings come from animal models and brain functional imaging like fMRI and PET research. These findings have resulted in the need for new approaches to the study of the Basal Ganglia from animal models to human brain mapping, translational and clinical practice, therefore, new interdisciplinary resources regarding Basal Ganglia are needed. All of the contributors to this volume have published in highly specialized research magazines but want to pioneer into a multidisciplinary open access work. This volume aims to provide online access to high-quality research and is an example of leading academics making their work visible and accessible to diverse audiences around the world.

Fernando A. Barrios and Clemens C. C. Bauer
Neurobiology Institute
National Autonomous University of Mexico,
Mexico

Chapter 1

Clinical Motor and Cognitive Neurobehavioral Relationships in the Basal Ganglia

Gerry Leisman, Robert Melillo and Frederick R. Carrick

Additional information is available at the end of the chapter

http://dx.doi.org/10.5772/55227

1. Introduction

The traditional view that the basal ganglia and cerebellum are simply involved in the control of movement has been challenged in recent years. One of the pivotal reasons for this reappraisal has been new information about basal ganglia and cerebellar connections with the cerebral cortex. In essence, recent anatomical studies have revealed that these connections are organized into discrete circuits or 'loops'. Rather than serving as a means for widespread cortical areas to gain access to the motor system, these loops reciprocally interconnect a large and diverse set of cerebral cortical areas with the basal ganglia and cerebellum. The properties of neurons within the basal ganglia or cerebellar components of these circuits resemble the properties of neurons within the cortical areas subserved by these loops. For example, neuronal activity within basal ganglia and cerebellar loops with motor areas of the cerebral cortex is highly correlated with parameters of movement, while neuronal activity within basal ganglia and cerebellar loops with areas of the prefrontal cortex is more related to aspects of cognitive function. Thus, individual loops appear to be involved in distinct behavioral functions. Studies of basal ganglia and cerebellar pathology support this conclusion. Damage to the basal ganglia or cerebellar components of circuits with motor areas of cortex leads to motor symptoms, whereas damage of the subcortical components of circuits with non-motor areas of cortex causes higher-order deficits. In this report, we review some of the new anatomical, physiological and behavioral findings that have contributed to a reappraisal of function concerning the basal ganglia and cerebellar loops with the cerebral cortex.

2. The basal ganglia in the context of behavior

The basal ganglia is part of a neuronal system that includes the thalamus, the cerebellum and the frontal lobes [1]. Like the cerebellum, the basal ganglion was previously thought to be primarily involved in motor control. However, recently there has been much written about and the role of the basal ganglia in motor and cognitive functions has now been well established [2-6].

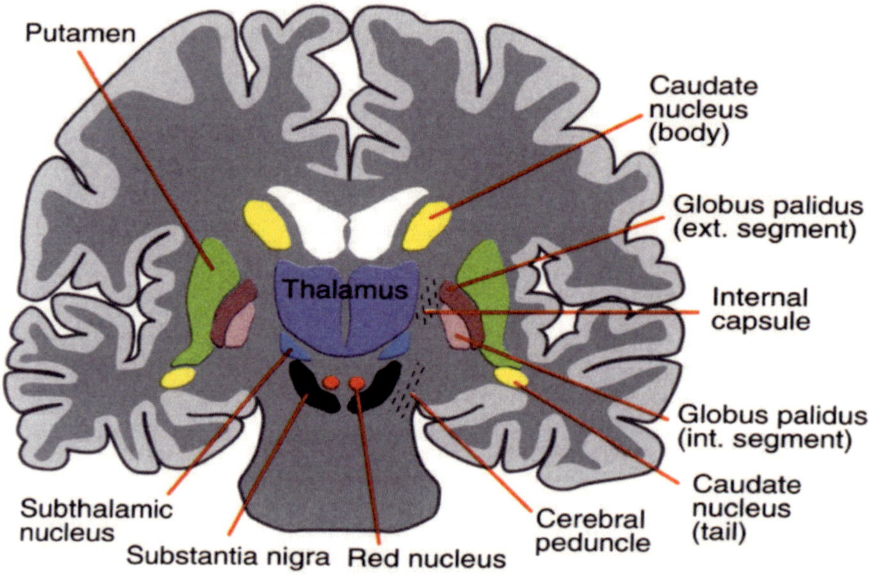

Figure 1. The basal ganglia that clinical include clinically includes subthalamic nucleus & substantia nigra whose component structures are highly interconnected. The striatum is associated with input signal and output associated with the globus pallidus & substantia nigra.

The basal ganglia is located in the diencephalon and is made up of five subcortical nuclei (represented in Fig.1): globus pallidus, caudate, putamen, substantia nigra and the subthalamic nucleus of Luys. The basal ganglia is thought to have expanded during the course of evolution as well and is therefore divided into the neo and paleostriatum. The paleostriatum consists primarily of the globus pallidus, which is derived embryologically from the diencephalon. During the course of its development it further divides into two distinct areas, the external and internal segments of the globus pallidus. The neostriatum is made up of two nuclei, the caudate and putamen. These two nuclei are fused anteriorly and are collectively known as the striatum. They are the input nuclei of the basal ganglia and they are derived embryologically from the telencephalon. The subthalamic nucleus of Luys lies inferiorly to the thalamus at the junction of the diencephalon and the mesencephalon or midbrain. The substantia nigra lays inferiorly to the thalamus and has two zones similar to the globus pallidus. A ventral pole zone called pars reticulata exists as well as a dorsal darkly pigmented zone called the pars compacta. The pars compacta contains dopaminergic neurons that contain the internum. The globus pallidus internum and the pars reticulata of the putamen are the major output nuclei of the basal ganglia. The globus pallidus internum and the pars reticulata of the putamen are similar in cytology, connectivity, and function. These two nuclei can be considered to be a single structure divided by the internal capsule. Their relationship is similar to that of the caudate and putamen. The basal ganglia is part of the extrapyramidal motor system as opposed to the pyramidal motor system that originates from the sensory-motor cerebral cortex. The pyramidal motor system is responsible for all voluntary motor activity except for eye movement. The extrapyramidal system modifies motor control and is thought to be involved with higher-order cognitive aspects of motor control as well as in the planning and execution of complex motor strategies, as well as the voluntary control of eye movements. There are two major pathways in the basal ganglia, the direct pathways, which promote movement, and the indirect pathways, which inhibit movement.

The basal ganglia receive afferent input from the entire cerebral cortex but especially from the frontal lobes. Almost all afferent connections to the basal ganglia terminate in the neostriatum (caudate and putamen). The neostriatum receives afferent input from two major sources outside of the basal ganglia, the cerebral cortex (cortico-striatal projections), and the intralaminar nucleus of the thalamus. The cortico- striatal projections contain topographically organized fibers originating from the entire cerebral cortex. An important component of that input comes from the centro-median nucleus from the thalamus and terminates in the putamen. Because the motor cortex of the frontal lobes projects to the centro-median nucleus, this may be an additional pathway by which the motor cortex can influence the basal ganglia. The putamen appears to be primarily concerned with motor control whereas the caudate appears to be involved in the control of eye movements and certain cognitive functions. The ventral striatum is related to limbic function, and therefore may affect autonomic and emotional functions.

The major output of the basal ganglia arises from the internal segment of the globus pallidus and the pars reticulata of the substantia nigra. The nuclei project in turn to three nuclei in the thalamus, the ventral lateral nuclei, the ventral anterior nuclei, and the mesio-dorsal nuclei, as well as the anterior thalamic nuclei. Internal segments of the globus pallidus project to the centro-median nucleus of the thalamus. Striatal neurons may be involved with gating incoming sensory input to higher motor areas such as the intralaminar thalamic nuclei and pre*motor* cortex that arise from several modalities to coordinate behavioral responses. These different modalities may contribute to the perception of sensory input [7] leading to motor response. The basal ganglia are directed, in a way similar to the cerebellum, to premotor and motor cortices as well as the prefrontal cortex of the frontal lobes.

Experiments where Herpes simplex virus 1 (HSV-1) was administered into the dorsal lateral prefrontal cortex of monkeys to determine its axonal spread or connection, labeled the ipsilateral neurons in the internal segments of the globus pallidus and the contralateral dentate nucleus of the cerebellum [8]. It is therefore thought that this may show a role of both the cerebellum and basal ganglia in higher cognitive functions associates with the prefrontal cortex. This would also substantiate a cortico-striato-cerebello-thalamo-cortical loop, which would have a cognitive rather than motor function, exemplified in Fig. 2 below. The putamen is also thought to connect to the superior colliculus through non-dopaminergic axons that forms an essential link in voluntary eye movement.

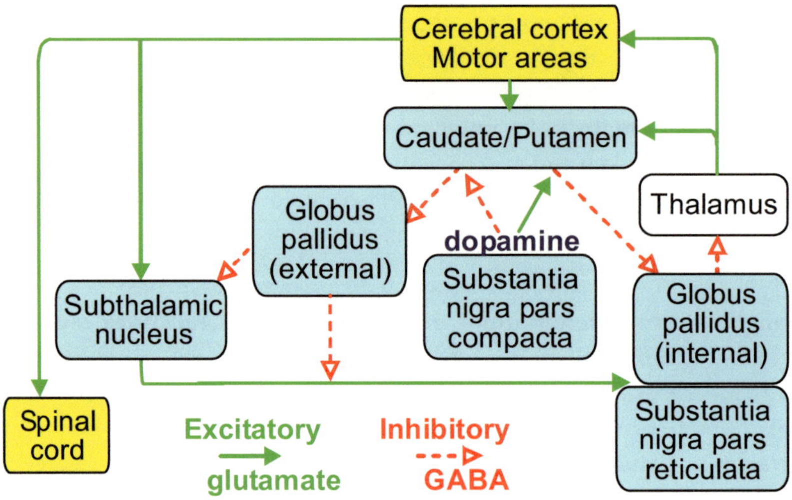

Figure 2. Circuitry of the basal ganglia. The cerebral cortex (and thalamus) projects to the striatum (excitatory pathways). The striatum also receives dopaminergic projections from the substania nigra's pars compacta (SNc). The striatum inhibits the globus pallidus (GP) as well as the substantia nigra's pars reticulata (SN pr). The STN sends excitatory projections to the GPi, GPe & SNpr. GPi or SN pr inhibits (GABAergic) the thalamus. The thalamus projects to the cortex (also excitatory). The direct path leads to less inhibition of the thalamus, (i.e. the striatum inhibits GPi which in turn inhibits its normal (inhibitory) action on the thalamus, thus leading to greater excitation from the thalamus to the cortex. This allows for sustain actions or initiation of action. The indirect path excites the GPi thereby increasing its inhibition of the thalamus and thus suppresses unwanted movements.

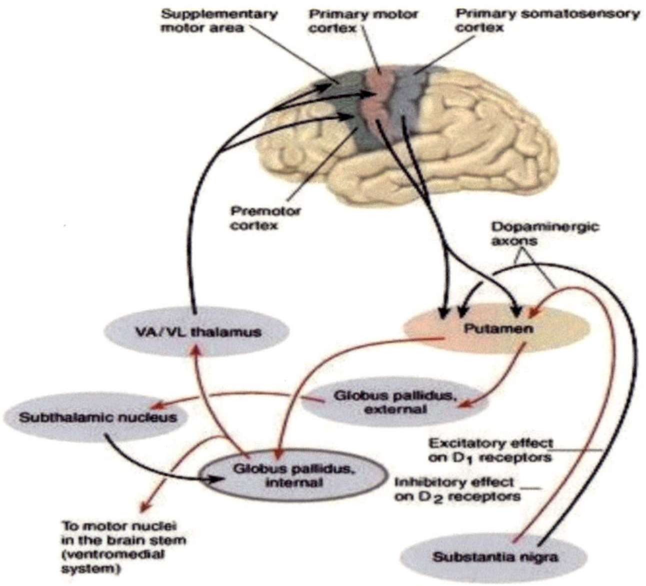

Figure 3. Cortical-basal ganglia pathways. All regions of cerebral cortex project to the basal ganglia, but output of basal ganglia is directed towards the frontal lobe, particularly pre-motor and supplementary motor cortex.

It is thought that normal basal ganglia function results from a balance of the direct and indirect striatal output pathway and different involvement of these pathways account for hyperkinesia or hypokinesia observed in disorders of the basal ganglia [9]. Hypokinesia is a disinhibition or increase in spontaneous movement (tics, tremors). It is thought that hypokinesia and hyperkinesia may relate to hypoactive behavior and hyperactive behavior associated with subcortical hypo-stimulation or hyper-stimulation of medial and orbito-frontal cortical circuits [10]. It is important to review these connections further to understand the role of basal ganglia in control of cognitive function.

Five fronto-subcortical circuits unite regions of the frontal lobe (the supplementary motor area; frontal eye fields; dorsolateral, prefrontal, orbito-frontal and anterior cingulate cortices) with the striatum, globus pallidus and thalamus in functional systems that mediate volitional motor activity, saccadic eye movements, executive functions, social behavior and motivation [10,11].

3. Direct and indirect pathways

Five major cortical to subcortical loops exist that make up cortico-striatal pathways. All cortical pathways initiate the direct and indirect pathways with the basal ganglia through excitatory glutamatergic cortico-striatal fibers (the general circuitry is described in Fig. 3 and direct and indirect pathways exemplified in Fig. 4). The direct pathway from the striatum sends GABA fibers (associated with dopamine receptors) from the striatum to the *globus pallidus* and putamen. The indirect pathway sends inhibitory GABA/enkephalin fibers (associated with D2 dopamine receptors) from the striatum to the globus pallidus. Indirect pathways then continue with inhibitory GABA fibers from the globus pallidus to the subthalamic nucleus of Luys. Indirect excitatory glutamatergic fibers then connect from the subthalamic nucleus to the globus pallidus and putamen. The basal ganglia then sends inhibitory outflow by GABA fibers from the globus pallidus and putamen to specific thalamic nuclei. The thalamus has excitatory fibers that return to the cortex [10]. Abnormalities of direct and indirect pathways result in different pathological functions.

The nature of the balance between components of these pathways is described in greater detail in the section below and described in Figs. 3-5. Hyperkinetic disorders (increased movement) are thought to be a selective loss of GABA/enkephalinergic intrinsic striatal neurons projecting to the lateral globus pallidus and substantia nigra. This results in decreased inhibitory stimulation to the thalamus leading to increased activity of the excitatory glutamatergic thalamocortical pathways and in turn greater neuronal activity in the premotor-motor and supplementary motor cortices [12]. The result is over-facilitation of motor programs resulting in increased motor activity. Hypokinetic disorders (decreased movement) are associated with decreased dopaminergic nigrostriatal stimulation from the substantia nigra to the striatum. This results in both excess outflow of the indirect striatal pathway and an inhibited direct striatal pathway. Both of these pathways increase thalamic inhibition and therefore decrease thalamocortical stimulation of motor cortical areas resulting in hypokinesia or decreased output of the frontal cortex [10,13,14]. It is possible

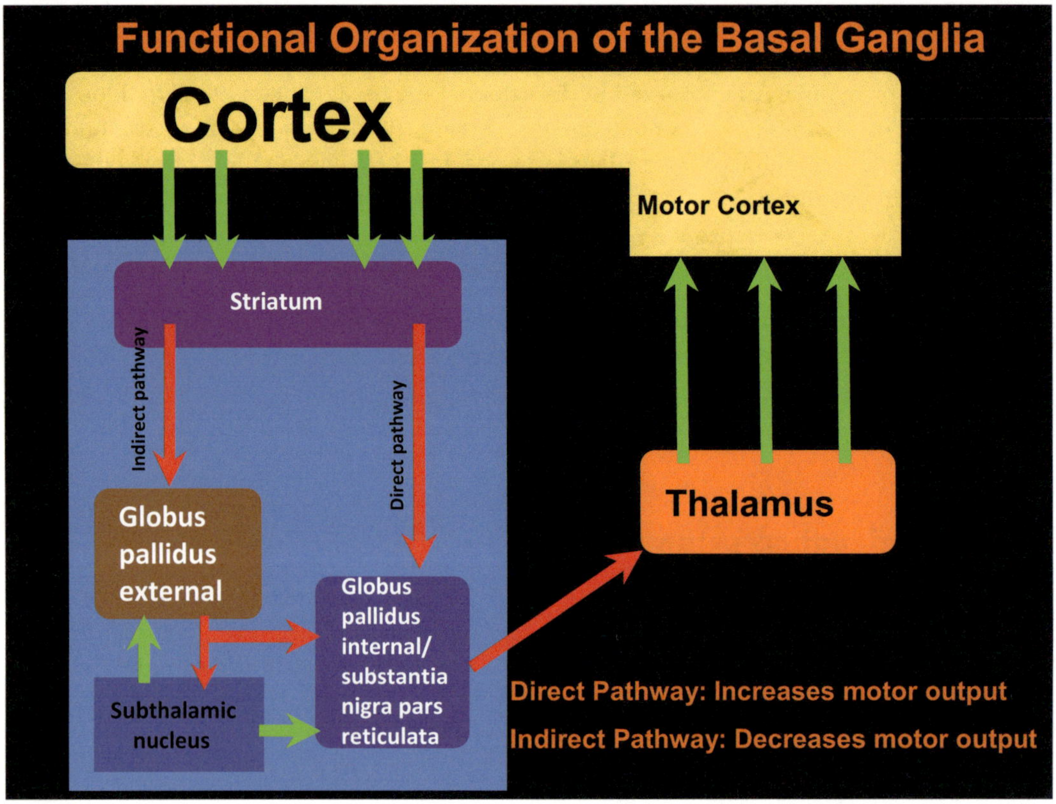

Figure 4. Direct and Indirect pathways. Direct pathway runs: Cortex→striatum→GPi→ thalamus→cortex. Two links are excitatory & two inhibitory, so the net effect of the whole sequence is excitatory. The cortex excites itself via the direct pathway. The Indirect pathway runs: cortex→striatum→GPe→ STN→Gpi→thalamus→cortex. Three links are inhibitory and two excitatory, so the net effect of the sequence is inhibitory: The cortex inhibits itself via the indirect pathway. The total effect of basal ganglia upon the cortex results from complex interplay between these two pathways.

that the difference between hypokinetic and hyperkinetic syndromes may be different only in the timing and or the severity of the dysfunction. In this model, decreased thalamic excitation of the frontal cortex results in decreased excitation of the cortico-striatal fibers of the neostriatum. The neostriatum therefore decreases its inhibitions of the globus pallidus. There is then increased inhibition of the thalamocortical pathways leading to progressive hypokinesia. Eventually the lack of striatal inhibition of the globus pallidus results in its metabolic dysfunction and the rapid loss of GABA neurons. This can then result in decreased inhibition of thalamocortical pathways causing a sudden onset of hyperkinesia (increased movement) with the increased thalamic firing of the frontal cortex. There also appear to exist cognitive symptoms that parallel the motor effects. Previous studies have shown that patients with hyperkinetic, hypokinetic, Tourette's, and Obsessive-Compulsive disorders may exhibit neuropsychiatric disturbances such as apathy, depression, agitation, or excitability [15-20].

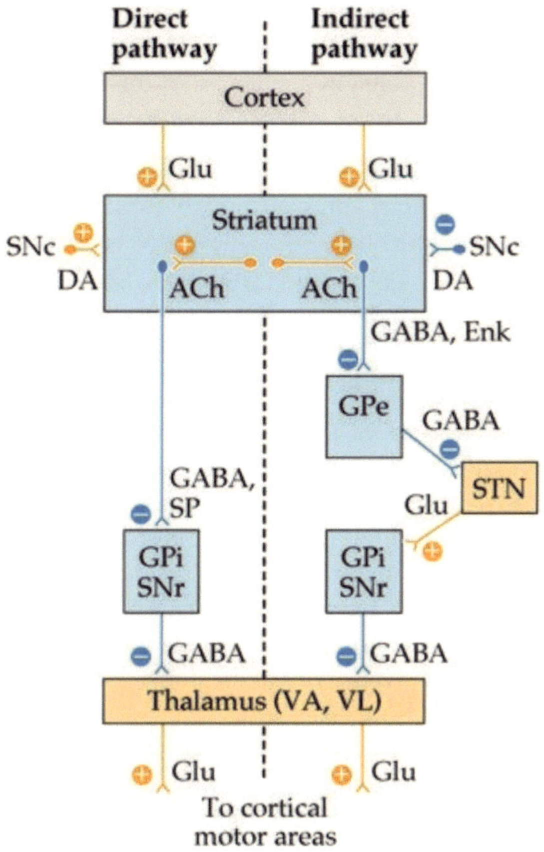

Figure 5. Circuit diagram for direct & indirect pathways. *Neurotransmitters:* Ach, acetylcholine; DA, dopamine; Glu, glutamate; Enk, enkaphalin; SP, substance P. *Nuclei:* SNc, substantia nigra pars compacta; SNr, substantia nigra pars retriculata; GPe, globus pallidus pars externa; GPi, globus pallidus pars interna; STN, subthalamic nucleus; VL, ventral lateral nucleus; VA, ventral anterior nucleus.

4. Clinical behavioral implications of pathway activity balance

Most disorders that involve the basal ganglia produce dysfunction by promoting an imbalance between the direct and indirect pathways. An increase in the relative activity in the direct pathways results in hyperkinetic movements and behaviors. This has been hypothesized to be a result of decreased activity of the indirect or increased activation of the direct pathway [11,13,14]. Increased relative activity in the indirect pathway is associated with hypokinetic movement and behaviors [21-23]. The majority of input to the basal ganglia comes from a top down direction through the five loops from the frontal lobe [24] referenced above. The premotor and supplementary motor areas, frontal and supplemental eye fields, the orbital frontal cortex, the dorsal lateral prefrontal cortex, and the anterior cingulate all connect into the basal ganglia governing voluntary motor activity, voluntary saccadic eye movement, social behavior, executive function, and motivation. These are then connected to various areas within the thalamus and back to the cortex. The indirect pathway increases the output of the globus pallidus internis [25,26] and increases the inhibition of the thalamus and motor activity or behaviors. Increase in direct pathway function inhibits the output of the globus pallidus thereby promoting increased movement and cognitive behaviors.

One of the main clinical questions especially in the absence of any obvious damage or pathology is what promotes a functional imbalance between these pathways (represented in Fig. 5). Various disorders such as ADHD, Tourette's, OCD among other are known to involve the basal ganglia. In these disorders there is hyperkinetic movement and or behaviors that coincide with the particular loop that is affected, but in all cases the increase seems to be in the direct loop not the indirect loop [9,11,17-21].

The principle question here is why these disorders would target an increase in this pathway in particular. One of the differences may have to do with the receptors that are involved in one pathway more than the other. The D1 receptor is known to be found in the direct pathway while the D2 receptor is found in the indirect loop. The nigrostriatal pathway is believed to help promote movement through its dopaminergic activity in the zona compacta by connecting to the Putamen and increasing the activity of the D1 receptor and inhibiting the D2 receptor [27]. Parkinson's Disease which is manifest as a hypokinetic disorder is, in part, related to this loss of increased activity to the direct pathway following degeneration of the dopaminergic neurons in the zona compacta. Using this as an example, other pathways that connect and enhance one receptor over the other is a way to functionally bias complementary pathways. We can understand the direct pathway as a behavioral activating pathway and the indirect as the behavioral inhibiting pathway [28]. This description can also been applied to the two cerebral hemispheres and their role in behavioral control. The left hemisphere is thought to promote approach behaviors [29,30], motor activity [24], intention [29] and positive emotions [30]. The right hemisphere is thought to promote withdrawal behavior [29], sensory and attentional activity [29], and negative affect [29]. The left hemisphere promotes motor and increases behavioral activity and motivation while the right hemisphere is known to do the opposite [29]. Therefore it is reasonable to assume that when utilizing top-down control, the two cerebral hemispheres may differentially enhance or inhibit motor activity and cognitive behavior.

The premotor areas and frontal eye fields increase volitional as well as involoutional motor activity and saccadic eye movements [31], the left orbital frontal cortex increases social motivation and awareness [29], the left dorsal lateral prefrontal cortex increases executive and cognitive function [24,30], while the left anterior cingulate increases motivation [29]. The right hemisphere decreases or inhibits those same pathways [32]. This would give even greater top-down control over these behaviors and it would make sense that this is done by enhancing the direct or indirect pathway.

The left hemisphere would promote and increase movement and behavior by selectively increasing the direct pathways perhaps by favoring the D1 receptors in the caudate and or putamen. The right hemisphere could promote the indirect pathway function by selectively enhancing or stimulating the D2 receptors in these same areas. Since many of the hyperkinetic disorders like ADHD, Tourette's and OCD have all been associated with a decreased function of the right hemisphere and an increased function of left hemisphere activity [24,33,34] that would also seem to fit with the argument that a decrease in right hemisphere function would be associated with an increase in left hemisphere function and enhancement of the direct pathway and the D1 receptor promoting hyperkinetic movement and behaviors.

The right hemisphere could also have stronger connections to the subthalamic nucleus of Luys which would also enhance the indirect pathway whereas stronger left hemisphere connections to the caudate and putamen may also enhance direct pathway activation over indirect [14]. There are other receptors that could be selectively targeted by one hemisphere more than the other. The hemispheres are well documented to have this type of differential top-down control over other functions such as the immune system [35], autonomic system [30] as well as top down control of sensory processing at the thalamic level with cortico-thalamic fibers outnumbering thalamocortical fibers by a 10 – 1 ratio [36].

The recent discovery of a hyperdirect pathway [37] confirms that this hemispheric relationship exists and in fact it seems to affect both pathways as we described. The right hemisphere generally is known to be more involved with behavioral inhibition whereas the left hemisphere generally is involved in behavioral excitation. This effect in part seems to be due to the relationship between the cortex, and the prefrontal cortex and basal ganglia. The five primary loops from the frontal lobe to the basal ganglia as we described include the premotor cortex for movement, the orbital frontal cortex for social behavior, the dorsolateral prefrontal cortex controls executive function, the anterior cingulate regulates motivation, and the frontal eye fields control saccadic eye movements. Together these loops help to regulate all human behaviors. The left hemisphere control appears to have an excitatory influence whereas the right hemisphere seems to subserve primarily an inhibitory control of these functions. This appears to mainly be accomplished by the hyperdirect pathway of the right hemisphere. The hyperdirect pathway accomplishes this through its influence on the D2 receptor which initiates the indirect pathway. This pathway increases the inhibitory output of the GPi and its influence on the thalamic relay nuclei.

The second way that the right hemisphere exerts this inhibitory control is through the hyperdirect connection from the inferior frontal gyrus directly through an excitatory glutamatenergic connection to the subthalamic nucleus of Luys. This increases the output of excitatory connections to the Gpi and an inhibitory connection to the GPe, which is inhibitory to the SNL. This also activates the indirect pathway increasing the inhibitory output of the GPi to the thalamus. Without this activity, the left hemisphere will have a relatively increased output to the D1 receptor activating the direct pathway, which decreases the output of the GPi through its inhibitory GABAnergic connections. This, in turn, decreases the inhibition of the thalamic nuclei thereby increasing activity in these prefrontal loops. The clinical implications of this are significant especially in functional lesions of the brain where there are no anatomic lesions but rather a primary imbalance between the direct and indirect pathways.

A functional imbalance and/or a functional disconnection between the two hemispheres, that may be the result of an activation imbalance in the cortex between the two hemispheres, can lead to an imbalance in these loops producing either hyperkinetic or hypokinetic disorders. This would explain why symptoms of hyperkinetic disorders like ADHD also seem to be associated with a decrease in many right hemisphere functions along with relative increases in left hemisphere functions. This also would mean that therapeutically increasing the activation through target stimulation to one hemisphere and possibly to one or more dysfunctioning basal ganglionic loops may help to restore a balance and temporal coherence between the hemispheres and between the direct and indirect loops.

For instance if someone is experiencing symptoms of OCD they have obsessions and compulsions in the absence of a specific lesion in the basal ganglia and specifically in the indirect pathway, this may be explained by decreased activation in the loops that involve the premotor cortex which control motor activity (compulsions) and the dorsolateral prefrontal cortex which controls executive functions, planning and behavior (obsessions) on the right hemisphere. This may result in a relative increase in those same loops on the left hemisphere leading to a relative increase of the direct pathway over the indirect pathway in those specific loops leading to OCD symptoms.

If this is the case then providing specific targeted stimulation to the premotor areas and the dorsolateral prefrontal cortex on the right hemisphere with the proper frequency, intensity and duration may produce an equilibration between the loops in those hemispheres and in the direct and indirect pathways. This may provide the best therapeutic option because it is specific, noninvasive and can provide long term correction which would be the ultimate goal.

5. Dynamic inter-regional effects

Disconnection syndromes were originally conceptualized as a disruption of communication between different cerebral cortical areas [30,31]. Schmahmann and Pandya [38] in an elegant review, indicate that the concept could be expanded. In overviewing their anatomical studies of monkeys, they found that efferent fibers emanate from every cortical area, and are directed with topographic precision via association fibers to ipsilateral cortical areas, commissural fibers to contralateral cerebral regions, striatal fibers to basal ganglia, and projection subcortical bundles to thalamus, brainstem and/or pontocerebellar system. They concluded that cortical areas are definable by their patterns of subcortical and cortical connections.

In applying their findings to humans, they note that motor, cognitive and neuropsychiatric disorders in patients with basal ganglia lesions, as well as those of the thalamus, or cerebellum, tend to mimic deficits resulting from cortical lesions, with qualitative differences between the manifestations of lesions in functionally related areas of cortical and subcortical nodes. These basal ganglia based behavioral conditions are viewed by Schmahmann and Pandya as disconnection syndromes reflecting loss of the contribution of subcortical nodes to the distributed neural circuits. They concluded that neural architecture determines function, i.e., each architectonically distinct cortical and subcortical area contributes a unique transform, or computation, to information processing as suggested by Leisman and Melillo [30]. Anatomically precise and segregated connections between nodes define behavior and association fiber tracts that link cerebral cortical areas with each other enable the cross-modal integration required for evolved complex behaviors.

Co-contration of muscle groups is realistically the co-activation of competing motor programs that serves as a fundamental mechanism used to achieve postural stabilization. Thus motor and cognitive signs associated with basal ganglionic lesions should also have a postural component that aids clinicians in the identification of lesions as well as providing a window for outcome observations when dealing with cognitive strategy efficacy.

The effective function involving the basal ganglia is traditionally thought to be achieved via a balance of excitation and inhibition of competing motor programs. In the context of this review, cognitive and motor functions need to be linked with postural control systems. These systems are known to be dynamic, rather than static. Hyperkinetic dystonias, for example, reflect excessive function of dynamic postures, rather than abnormal movements. Anne Blood [39] has suggested that the range of functional roles served by the postural system is hypothesized to include direct control of movement, suggesting a postural basis for task-specific dystonias. Further, by defining posture as a neural system that maintains body stabilization, it can be shown that the range of mechanical means of implementing stabilization, including co-contraction of antagonistic muscles, matches the range of presentations of dystonia reflecting abnormal integration in the basal ganglia. Inhibitory influences that stabilizing mechanisms exert on movement, suggest that the broad functional role of posture may be the function served by the indirect pathway of the basal ganglia. Specifically, the integrated pathway that centrally coordinates function of the distributed network of brain regions controlling posture and, in conjunction with the direct pathway, coordinates posture and movement. Postural systems are probably involved in cognition as well as the motor volitional and reflexogenic parameters of basal ganglionic influence. The involvement of posture in the basal ganglia and behavioral relationships is further supported by Marsden and Rothwell [41] who noted that co-contraction is realistically the co-activation of competing motor programs that serves as a fundamental mechanism used to achieve postural stabilization.

Numerous other investigators have recently begun to notice the relationship of posture to basal ganglia and cognitive function serving as a basis for the clinical discussions in the subsequent section. Mitra and colleagues [40] noted that the performance of a cognitive task while maintaining upright stance is associated with changes in body sway depending on tasks and experimental conditions. As increased sway is taken to indicate loosened postural control the precise impact of cognitive load on postural stability has remained unclear. These investigators noted that body sway increased during cognitive tasks while quiet standing but not while performing a visuo-postural alignment task suggesting that constraints placed on posture control by supra-postural task goals may significantly alter interactions between posture control and cognitive task.

Fujiwara and associates [42] investigated the effect of neck flexion on discriminative and cognitive processing in postural control during bilateral arm movement while standing, using event-related potential (ERP) and electromyogram. They noted significant positive correlations with neck flexion and P3 latency and anterior deltoid reaction time, and between N2 latency and the onset time of erector spinae, suggesting that with neck flexion, attention allocation to discriminative and cognitive processing increases, and the processing speed increases with shortening of reaction time in focal muscles.

Thus there is enough preliminary evidence to indicate that motor and cognitive signs associated with basal ganglionic lesions should also have a postural component that would aid clinicians in the identification of lesions as well as providing a window for outcome observations when dealing with cognitive strategy efficacy.

6. Clinical implications

It has been hypothesized that neuropsychiatric symptoms exhibited by patients with basal ganglia disorders are a consequence of an involvement of fronto-striatal connections. In addition to expressing contrasting motor dysfunction patterns, these disorders would also differ in the presenting psychiatric symptoms [10]. In this study patients with Huntington's disease (hyperkinetic) and Parkinson's disorder (hypokinetic) were observed to determine if they would present with hyperactive behavior (agitation, isolation, euphoria, or anxiety) and hypokinetic behavior (apathy) respectively. The results of this study demonstrated that patients with Huntington's (hyperkinetic) more frequently exhibited hyperactive behaviors such as agitation, irritability, euphoria, and anxiety whereas patients with Parkinson's (hypokinetic) frequently displayed hypoactive behavior (high levels of apathy). The investigators thought that in Huntington's, these behaviors result from excitatory subcortical output through the medial and orbito-frontal circuits to the pallidum, thalamus, and cortex as well as premotor and motor cortex. In contrast, patients with Parkinson's (hypoactive) in whom apathy is present were thought to demonstrate these behaviors as a consequence of hypo-stimulation of frontal subcortical circuits resulting from damage to several integrated nuclei (putamen, striatum and globus pallidus) [14,43,44].

It had been previously noted that patients with Huntington's and other hyperkinetic disorders like Tourette's exhibit mania, OCD, and intermittent explosive disorder [45,46-48]. PET studies of Huntington's patients without hyperactive behavior have shown frontal metabolism to be normal but with decreased caudate and putamen metabolism [49,50]. However is it thought that normal frontal metabolism in Huntington's may result from a coexistent neurological degeneration and the resultant thalamo-frontal hyper-stimulation. This may result in normal appearing frontal-cortical regional blood flow even when overt prefrontal type cognitive defects are manifested. This suggests that in this case, a dysfunctional prefrontal cortex may appear to be at baseline levels that appear normal when in fact the prefrontal cortices may be over stimulated by the thalamus. [51,52]. In fact, it was noted that with further atrophy of the caudate there was increased fronto-cortical metabolism while the patient performed cognitive tasks (set-shifting) and a greater increase in cerebral metabolism over baseline. The poorer the subject performed on cognitive tasks, the greater the cortical activation. [51,52]. It has been speculated that in early Huntington's when there are no frontal lobe lesions, a relative balance between frontal and increased thalamic functions may explain behavioral symptoms [10].

PET scans of patients with Parkinson's have also provided support that frontal-subcortical connections are disrupted by subcortical dysfunction showing decreased glucose consumption in frontal cortex, and decrease nigrostriatal D2 receptor uptake ratios [53,54]. Researchers at Stanford University may have observed similar results in children with *ADHD* also known as childhood hyperkinetic disorder [55]. The Stanford study used functional MRI to image the brains of boys between the ages of 8 and 13 while playing a mental game. Ten of the boys were diagnosed with *ADHD* and six were considered normal. When the boys were tested there appeared to be a clear difference in the activity of the basal ganglia with the boys with *ADHD* having less activity in that area than the control subjects. After administering methylphenidate, the participants were scanned again and it was found that boys with *ADHD* had increased activity in the basal ganglia whereas the normal boys had decreased activity in the basal ganglia. Interestingly, the drug improved the performance of both groups to the same extent.

This may be a similar finding as the PET scans on patients with hyperactivity disorder, where normal appearing frontal metabolism existed with decreased caudate and putamen metabolism [56]. Methylphenidate, a dopamine reuptake inhibitor, may increase function in a previously dysfunctional basal ganglia whereas raising dopamine levels in normal individuals would most likely result in decreased activity of the basal ganglia to prevent overproduction of dopamine. The previously dysfunctional basal ganglia would have most likely resulted in decreased frontal metabolism with increased thalamo-cortical firing; this would result in decreased cognitive function with increased hyperkinetic (hyperactive) behavior. Increasing dopamine levels may increase frontal metabolism due to increased activity of the striatum with decreased firing of the globus pallidus thereby inhibiting thalamo-cortical firing decreases which in turn decreases hyperkinetic behavior. This would make sense based on the findings of fMRI before and after, and the fact that both groups showed equal improvement in performance.

7. Basal ganglia in obsessive compulsive disorder

Cognitive and brain maturational changes continue throughout late childhood and adolescence. During this time, increasing cognitive control over behavior enhances the voluntary suppression of reflexive/impulsive response tendencies [29,30]. We presently have the capacity to characterize changes in brain activity during cognitive development. Optimized top-down modulation of the ability to voluntarily suppress context-inappropriate behavior of reflexive acts is not fully developed until adulthood and this process provides a context to examine the nature of obsessive-compulsive disorder in a maturational context and within the framework of the basal ganglia and its networks.

The basal ganglia-thalamo-cortical circuits appear to play a modulating role in a wide range of behaviors. At the cortical level, given convergence upon specified regions within the frontal lobes, the behaviors in question would be those dependent upon the sensory-motor, premotor, frontal eye fields, and dorsolateral and orbito-frontal outflow targets. Processes such as the generation, maintenance, switching, and blending of motor, mental, or emotional sets would be involved. In disorders that primarily affect basal ganglia function, the planning and the execution of both motor and cognitive function within these behavioral domains could be affected. As we have seen, there is a high degree of diversity and complexity of activity within the basal ganglia. Despite the nature of the reverberating circuits, consequences of disruption will depend upon the site of the lesion and the associated interplay of neurochemical factors. For example, in the motor system, damage to various striatal circuitry levels can result in either hypo- or hyperkinetic disorders of movement. Following this analogy, it can be said that diverse lesions, depending on site, can result in problems with the development and maintenance of behavioral sets ("hypophrenic") versus problems in relinquishing preferential sets ("hyperphrenic"). In OCD, a "hyperphrenic" pattern would apply to those behaviors which are part of obsessional rituals.

There is evidence of basal ganglia dysfunction from imaging studies of OCD, with both reduced and increased volumes of caudate nuclei reported [57-59]. Increased caudate metabolism has been found to be reduced after effective treatment of the OCD [60,61 and in provoked or activated conditions, patients with OCD have shown increased caudate blood flow [62. Such imaging studies point to the importance of orbito-frontal-basal ganglia-thalamocortical circuits in the pathogenesis of OCD. In autism stereotyped, ritualistic and repetitive behaviors including compulsive rituals and difficulties in tolerating changes in routine or environment, are characteristic. It has been suggested [24,63,64] that these behaviors may share related pathophysiological mechanisms. Sears and colleagues [63] analyzed with high resolution MRI the volume of the bilateral caudate, putamen, and globus pallidus regions in a group with autism and a control group. No differences were detected in volumes of the globus pallidus or the putamen. Significant enlargement of 8 percent of the total caudate volume was found in the subjects with autism. This greater caudate volume was proportional to the increased total brain volume and enlargement of other brain structures earlier reported in the patients with autism. [65].

Based on the aforementioned studies and the basis of this chapter, the cortico-basal ganglia circuits linking the orbito-frontal and anterior cingulate cortex to the caudate nucleus might account for the cardinal features of OCD. All of these structures have been implicated in the evaluation of the significance of stimulating as positive or negative (rewarding or punishing) and all, as we have seen, have been linked to aspects of executive function. Cortical-basal ganglia circuits have been suggested to form a neuronal system critical for habit learning and for the routine performance of habits, and structures of the OCD circuit have specifically been implicated in the acquisition of stereotyped behaviors [66,67].

The basal ganglia are thought to exert control over action release through antagonistic "push-pull" output pathways, which serve to select intended actions [68]. As explained earlier in the chapter, these functions are disrupted in hypokinetic disorders such as Parkinson's disease, in which action is diminished, and in the hyperkinetic disorders such as in Huntington's disease, in which action is excessive. Analogously, it has been suggested that the function of these cortico-basal ganglia pathways may also occur in some neuropsychiatric disorders including OCD and Tourette's syndrome.

Different sets of cortical-basal ganglia loops are thought to have specialized functions depending on the cortical areas participating in the loops. This organization may account for the symptom specificity of OCD as compared to other disorders of the basal ganglia and its pathways. For example, in Tourette's syndrome, in which the characteristics of actions are the predominant symptoms, the "motor loop" through the putamen is more effective than it is in OCD according to neuroimaging data [69-71]. In OCD, which typically involves obsessions as well as compulsive actions, the neuronal circuits interconnecting the orbito-frontal and anterior cingulate cortex with the basal ganglia are involved.

The caudate nucleus has been implicated in repetitive actions in monkeys. The orbital-frontal and the anterior cingulate cortex both project to the ventral part of the caudate nucleus and to the ventral striatum. In the monkey, these regions have been found to send outputs not only to the pallidum, but also to a large part of the dopamine-containing substantia nigra pars compacta, from which the nigro-striatal tract originates. The caudal orbito-frontal and anterior cingulate/caudal medial cortex are also a major source of input to the striosomal system in the head of the caudate nucleus. Striosomes in this region have been linked to reward effects and may appear to be differentially active under conditions in which the animals perform repetitive, stereotyped behaviors in response to dopamine receptor agonists [72].

These features of the orbito-frontal and anterior cingulate cortical-basal ganglia circuits are important not only for understanding OCD symptomatology, but also for understanding the developmental aspects of these disorders. The basal ganglia may influence of motor pattern generators in the brainstem as well as "cognitive pattern generators" in the cerebral cortex. The loops running from the neocortex to the basal ganglia and then to the thalamus and back to the neocortex may help to establish cognitive habits, just as they may influence the development of motor habits. If so, the cortical-basal ganglia loop dysfunction in OCD could reflect both sides of basal ganglia function, motor and cognitive, to bring about repetitive actions (compulsions) and repetitive thoughts (obsessions).

Alternatively, the basal ganglia may have as its task a process that takes input form cortical and other sources and releases the output as "chunks" in order to sequence behavior, important in forming coordinated, sequential motor actions and in developing streams of thoughts and motivation, and perhaps playing the violin [63]. The architecture of cortical-basal ganglia circuitry could support the smooth progression from a cognitive framework establishing priorities for potential behaviors to behavioral selection, thereby facilitating fluid and adaptive behavioral output. Dysfunction of this cortical-basal ganglia system could contribute to the symptoms of OCD. Individuals become stuck in a conceptual framework, unable to shift from one priority set to the next, and thus remain locked into a specific behavioral output program.

A large part of the frontal cortex receives inputs from the basal ganglia conveyed via the thalamus. These same cortical regions not only project to the basal ganglia (mainly to the striatum) but also to other regions including the thalamus. Cortical-thalamic loops are critical for integrative and optimized cortical functioning. The adequacy of basal ganglia function is necessary to facilitate associations among cortical inputs on the basis of context and evaluative signals, and thereby promote behavioral automation, normally necessary to reduce the information load on the system. The basal ganglia can relieve the frontal cortex of the substantial computational load in carrying out executive functions. With both cortical-thalamic and cortical-basal ganglia systems functioning under normal conditions, parallel processing can occur with the cortical-thalamic circuits supporting conscious (explicit) information processing and cortical-basal ganglia supporting automatic (implicit) processing functions. If cortical-basal ganglia pathways functional abnormally, as in OCD such parallel processing capabilities would be compromised. Information normally processed automatically could intrude into the conscious domain of sessions, and behavioral selection could become narrowed to compulsive acts. Such dysfunction could contribute to the compelling nature of obsessions in OCD and to the stereotypic behaviors carried out as compulsions.

The cortical-basal ganglia circuits appear dysfunctional in OCD, but the mechanisms are not adequately understood at present. While we have seen that striatal lesions can induce intense compulsive behaviors and stereotypies, we have not as yet found the existence of subtle lesions of the striatum in OCD, perhaps as a result of the inadequacies of our current measuring instruments. Magnetic resonance spectroscopy studies have suggested that there exists reduced N-acetylaspartate levels within the striatum of persons with OCD, so that neuronal density there may actually be reduced [17,74. Abnormal brain chemistry in OCD could affect neurotransmission in cortical-basal ganglia circuits leading to the abnormal metabolic activity seen in imaging studies indicated earlier. While little is known about neurochemistry of OCD, the most successful pharmacologic therapy for OCD is treatment with inhibitors of serotonin reuptake (SRIs) sites. Effective therapy with SRIs can reverse the abnormal metabolic activity seen in OCD circuits, suggesting that the modulatory effects of serotonin can act on the cortical-basal ganglia circuit defined in scanning studies [75].

Despite the clinical results, strong evidence of a primary serotonergic or other neurotransmitter abnormality in OCD is still lacking. One suggestion is that SRIs have their beneficial effects via downregulation of 5HT-1D autoreceptors within the orbito-frontal cortex [75]. Even though neuroimaging studies have pointed to cortico-basal ganglia circuits as being dysfunctional in OCD, it is still not clear what the functional abnormality is in the circuits in OCD and how they contribute to the expression of OCD symptoms. Nor is it clear how these circuits were normally, or help multiple loops of the system interconnecting cortex, thalamus, and basal ganglia actually operate. Improvements in the temporal and spatial resolution of imaging also now make it possible to follow the cascade of neuronal activity changes that occur during the evolution of OCD symptoms. It should be possible in the relatively near future to identify brain sites participating in the buildup of an obsession, the attendant anxiety, the escalation of an urge, the performance of a compulsion, and the resolution of the obsession and accompanying anxiety.

8. Basal ganglia in tourette's syndrome

Tourette's syndrome (TS) is a neurobehavioral disorder characterized by involuntary motor and vocal tics beginning in childhood [76]. Approximately 50 percent of individuals with TS also exhibit obsessive–compulsive disorder (OCD) in addition; tics and OCD individuals demonstrate similar features and both are thought to arise from frontal-cortical–basal ganglia–thalamo–cortical circuit dysfunction. Recent advances in understanding the neurobiology of TS come from neuroimaging, post-mortem, and from physiological and behavioral studies in human and non-human primates and rodents. These advances allow us to understand the nature of the complex dynamics of the basal ganglia pathways and how this disorder connects with other forms of cognitive dysfunction.

Tourette's syndrome is defined by motor and vocal tics that start during childhood, persist for more than one year, and fluctuate in type, frequency and anatomical distribution over time. A specific tic can be present for weeks, months or years and then suddenly cease. Other tics emerge and disappear with no predictable time course. The motor patterns of tics can involve individual muscles or small groups of muscles (simple tics), or more muscles acting in a coordinated pattern to produce movements that can resemble purposeful voluntary movements (complex tics). Many individuals with TS exhibit both simple and complex tics. Simple tics include eye blinking, nose twitching, head jerking, eye deviation, mouth opening, sniffing and throat clearing. Complex tics include head shaking, scratching, touching, throwing, hitting, gestures or uttering phrases. There is a tendency for tics to occur in 'bouts' that wax and wane over hours, days, weeks or months [77].

OCD is strongly associated with TS both within individuals with TS and within families [78]. As indicated above, OCD is characterized by repetitive thoughts that are involuntary, senseless and often associated with anxiety, coupled with repetitive ritualistic behaviors that are often performed in response to the premonitory thought or idea. There are striking similarities between tics and OCD, and it is sometimes difficult to distinguish complex tics from compulsions. Both tics and OCD include premonitory experiences such as sensations (tics) or thoughts (OCD) that precede involuntary repetitive movements (tics) or behaviors (OCD). Performance of the tic or compulsion typically terminates the premonitory symptoms, at least temporarily.

Another feature common to both phenomena but important for placing OCD and Tourette's within the cortico-basal ganglia loop process, is the impaired ability each disorder to inhibit unwanted actions [79,80]. The spectrum of simple tics, complex tics, and compulsions suggests that similar or shared pathophysiological mechanisms, but separate neural circuits, might underlie these phenomena. These overlaps can be seen in cases of poisoning especially with carbon monoxide in which the basal ganglia is selectively affected and symptoms have been reported not dissimilar from those of Tourette's syndrome [79].

It is useful for us to examine cursorily issues related the neuropharmacology of TS to better understand the nature of the loops and the connection of TS to OCD. Tics are suppressed reliably by dopamine antagonists and OCD is improved by selective serotonin-reuptake inhibitors (SSRIs) [81]. These facts implicate the dopaminergic and serotonergic pathways and suggest the candidate loci for TS abnormalities. The implicated regions include the striatum, the substantia nigra, and the prefrontal cortices. The dopaminergic complex of the substantia nigra and ventral tegmental area and the serotonergic dorsal raphé nuclei both send major projections to the striatum. The striatum, prefrontal cortices and substantia nigra are further interlinked by a web of pathways that form the cortical–basal ganglia–thalamo–cortical circuits [82-85].

We can infer from the literature cited previously that TS is a disorder of the basal ganglia and its respective pathways in general, and a disorder of striatal organization and/or function in particular. Some correlative data from other disorders supports the idea that striatal dysfunction is involved in TS. Tics are seen also in disorders with known striatal pathology, such as Huntington's disease [21,76]. Abundant data implicates ventral striatal dopaminergic neurotransmission in drug abuse and drug craving, attributes of which overlap with obsessive–compulsive disorder (OCD) [86].

The clinical presentation of TS should reflect involvement of striatal function. Tics, in general, are abnormal repetitive and stereotyped movements, but repetitive stereotyped behaviors also occur normally. These behavioral effects are consistent with the effects of D1 receptor agonists on the response of medium spiny striatal neurons to stimulation [87]. D1 agonists tend to potentiate the current state of striatal neurons and reinforce ongoing behaviors. The complex and perseverative behaviors caused by D1 agonists differ from the effects of D2 receptor agonists, which tend to cause simple repetitive stereotyped movements. Kelly and Berridge [86] suggest that super-stereotypy is analogous to complex tics or OCD. Other stereotyped behavioral sequences are modulated by the basal ganglia include complex defensive behaviors and facial movements.

Charles Darwin [88] had indicated that many facial movements are stereotyped among mammals and important in non-verbal communication. Because tics commonly involve involuntary head, neck and face movements, the importance of facial and related movements in social communication might explain the disruptive nature of tics. There are suggestions that regulation of socially relevant forms of communication is a phylogenetically ancient function of the basal ganglia.

Additionally, the basal ganglia participate in brain circuits responsible for habit formation and fixed action patterns [29]. Habits are physiological analogs of stereotyped, unconsciously executed behavioral sequences such as tics, obsessions and compulsions. The basal ganglia participate in circuits responsible for learning incremental stimulus–response associations epitomized by classical Pavlovian and instrumental conditioning [89]. Graybiel has emphasized that the basal ganglia might combine or 'chunk' individual stimulus–response associations into more complex behavioral sequences executed as stereotyped 'units' as we had seen earlier [68]. In addition, fMRI study of higher-order aversive conditioning, in which key computational strategy that humans use to learn predictions about pain was investigated. The investigators showed that neural activity in the ventral striatum and the anterior insula display marked correspondence to the signals for sequential learning predicted by temporal difference models. They identified the ventral striatum as a key locus of such sequential learning [90]. Tics could represent a form of inappropriate habit formation in which inappropriate stimulus–response associations are formed. This interpretation might correlate with the fluctuating nature and 'sensory' component of tics.

In the study of non-human primates, electrophysiological studies of the intralaminar thalamic nuclei have revealed that these nuclei influence striatal attentional mechanisms and the processing of reward information [91]. These studies also suggest that intralaminar thalamic nuclei encode information complementary to the reward prediction error information provided by the dopaminergic nigrostriatal projection.

Basal ganglia circuitry models that we had described earlier in the paper view the normal, tonically active inhibitory output of the basal ganglia as a 'brake' on motor pattern generators (MPGs) in the cerebral cortex and brainstem [92]. For a desired movement controlled by a particular MPG, a specific set of striatal neurons is activated; these neurons inhibit basal ganglia output neurons in the GPi and substantia nigra pars reticulata (SNr) that project back, via the thalamus, to the cortical MPGs. The removal of tonic inhibition from the GPi and SNr (the 'brake') enables the desired motor pattern to proceed. In parallel, neurons in the subthalamic nucleus (STN) excite the surrounding majority of GPi and SNr output neurons. These surround neurons project via the thalamus to competing MPGs, increasing their inhibitory output and applying the "brake" to competing MPGs. The net result is facilitation of intended movement with inhibition of competing movements. In the generation of tics, it is hypothesized that an aberrant focus of striatal neurons becomes inappropriately active, causing unwanted inhibition of a group of basal ganglia output neurons, which in turn disinhibit an MPG leading to an involuntary movement. Repetitive over-activity of a given specific set of striatal neurons would result in repeated, stereotyped, unwanted movements [92]. Multiple tics would result from abnormal excessive activity of multiple discrete sets of striatal neurons According to this hypothesis, each tic corresponds to the activity of a discrete set of striatal neurons [79].

9. Basal ganglia in ADHD

Attention-deficit/hyperactivity disorder is a highly heritable and prevalent neuropsychiatric disorder estimated to affect six percent of school-age children [24]. It is manifested by inattention, hyperactivity and impulsivity, which often respond substantially to treatment with methylphenidate or dextroamphetamine. Etiological theories suggest a deficit in cortico-striatal circuits, particularly those components modulated by dopamine and therefore discussed in comparison with the other basal ganglia related disorders in the paper. Teicher and colleagues [94] developed a functional magnetic resonance imaging procedure (T2 relaxometry) to indirectly assess blood volume in the striatum (caudate and putamen) of boys 6–12 years of age in steady-state conditions. Boys with attention-deficit/hyperactivity disorder had higher T2 relaxation time measures in the putamen bilaterally than healthy control subjects. Daily treatment with methylphenidate significantly changed the T2 relaxation times in the putamen of children with attention deficit/

hyperactivity disorder. There was a similar but non-significant trend in the right caudate. Teicher and colleagues concluded that attention-deficit/hyperactivity disorder symptoms may be closely tied to functional abnormalities in the putamen, which is mainly involved in the regulation of motor behavior.

Converging evidence implies the involvement of dopaminergic fronto-striatal circuitry in ADHD. Anatomical imaging studies using MRI have demonstrated subtle reductions in volume in regions of the basal ganglia and prefrontal cortex [e.g., 95]. Cognitive functioning is mildly impaired in this disorder [for review, see 90]. In particular, cognitive control, the ability to inhibit inappropriate thoughts and actions, is also affected and therefore we are again dealing with a disorder of inhibition. Several studies have shown that this impairment is related to the reduction in volume in fronto-striatal regions [96], and functional studies have suggested that older children and adults with ADHD may activate these regions less than controls during tasks that require cognitive control [e.g. 98, 99]. Durston et al. [100] showed that the development of this ability is related to the maturation of ventral fronto-striatal circuitry.

Volumetric abnormalities have also been associated with the basal ganglia and in turn with attention deficit hyperactivity disorder (ADHD). Qiu and colleagues [101], to specify localization of these abnormalities, employed large deformation diffeomorphic metric mapping (LDDMM) to examine the effects of ADHD, sex, and their interaction on basal ganglia shapes. The basal ganglia (caudate, putamen, globus pallidus) were manually delineated on magnetic resonance imaging from typically developing children and children with ADHD. LDDMM mappings from 35 typically developing children were used to generate basal ganglia templates. These investigators found that boys with ADHD showed significantly smaller basal ganglia volumes compared with typically developing boys, and LDDMM revealed the groups remarkably differed in basal ganglia shapes. Volume compression was seen bilaterally in the caudate head and body and anterior putamen as well as in the left anterior globus pallidus and right ventral putamen. Volume expansion was most pronounced in the posterior putamen. They concluded that the shape compression pattern of basal ganglia in ADHD suggests an atypical brain development involving multiple frontal-subcortical control loops, including circuits with premotor, oculomotor, and prefrontal cortices.

Aron and colleagues [102] brilliantly outlined the nature of inhibition in fronto-basal-ganglia networks relative to cognition. Their paper was not about the problems of ADHD individuals per se but a thorough analysis of the neurophysiology of stopping. They hand indicated that sensory information about a stop signal is relayed to the prefrontal cortex, where the stopping command must be generated. They collected the evidence together indicating that the right inferior frontal cortex (IFC) is a critical region for stop signal response inhibition [103,104] with the most critical portion likely being the pars opercularis (Brodmann area 44) in humans. The right IFC can send a stop command to intercept the Go process via the basal ganglia (represented in Fig. 6b from Aron et al., [102]. The Go process is likely generated by premotor areas that project via the direct pathway of the basal ganglia (through striatum, pallidum, and thalamus), eventually exciting primary motor cortex and generating cortico-spinal volleys to the relevant effector each interacting with the globus pallidus [105]. The Stop process could activate the globus pallidus via a projection from the subthalamic nucleus (STN). High resolution fMRI has shown activation of a midbrain region, consistent with the STN, when subjects successfully stop their responses [105], and diffusion tractography shows that this STN region is directly connected to the right IFC via a white matter tract [102] (Fig. 6c). Thus, once the Stop command is generated in frontal cortex, it could be rapidly conveyed to the basal ganglia via the so-called "hyperdirect pathway" to intercept the Go process in the final stages of the race. Two recent studies identified a third critical node for the stopping process in the dorso-medial frontal cortex, including the pre-supplementary motor area) [106,107].

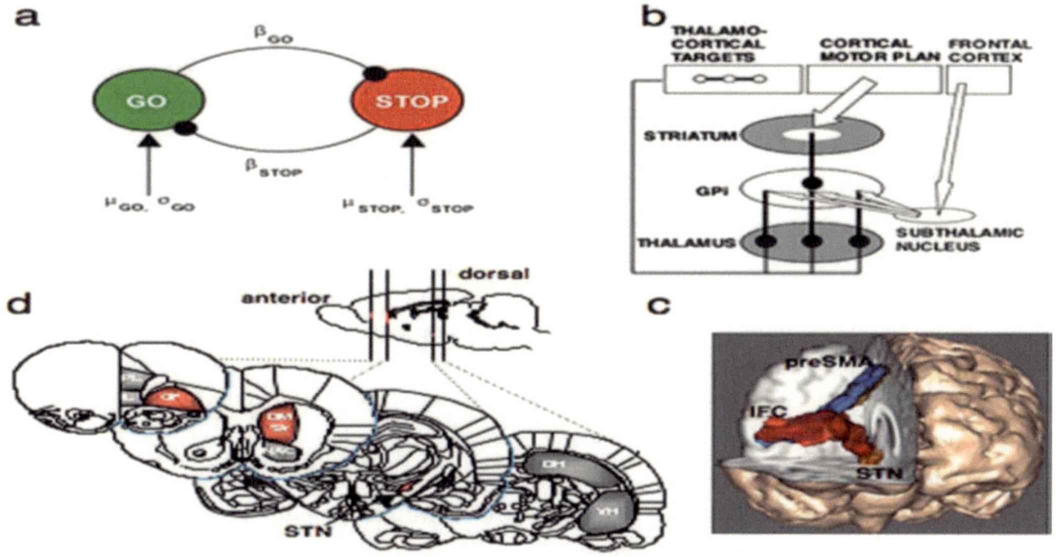

Figure 6. A, The interactive race model between Go and Stop processes [108]. The parameters were estimated by fitting the model to thousands of behavioral trials from a monkey neurophysiology study.B, Schematic of fronto-basal-ganglia circuitry for Going and Stopping. The Go process is generated by premotor cortex, which excites striatum and inhibits globus pallidus, removing inhibition from thalamus and exciting motor cortex (see text for details). The stopping process could be generated by inferior frontal cortex leading to activation of the subthalamic nucleus, increasing broad excitation of pallidum and inhibiting thalamocortical output, reducing activation in motor cortex. C, Diffusion-weighted imaging reveals putative white matter tracts in the right hemisphere between the dorsomedial preSMA, the ventrolateral PFC or IFC, and the putative region of the STN. Reproduced with permission from Aron et al. [102]. *D*, Regions of the rat brain implicated in behavioral stopping. Stopping is significantly impaired following excitotoxic lesions within the regions highlighted in red, whereas lesions within the gray-colored regions have no effect on stopping. OF, Orbitofrontal cortex; IL, infralimbic cortex; PL, prelimbic cortex; DM Str, dorsomedial striatum; NAC, nucleus accumbens (core); DH, dorsal hippocampus; VH, ventral hippocampus; GPi, globus pallidus pars interna. (From Aron et al. [102]),

10. Conclusions

Neural circuits linking activity in anatomically segregated populations of neurons in subcortical structures and the neocortex throughout the human brain regulate complex behaviors such as walking, talking, language comprehension and other cognitive functions including those associated with frontal lobes. Many neocortical and subcortical regions support the cortical-striatal-cortical circuits that confer various aspects of language ability, for example. However, many of these structures also form part of the neural circuits regulating other aspects of behavior. For example, the basal ganglia, which regulate motor control, are also crucial elements in the circuits that confer human linguistic ability and reasoning. The cerebellum, traditionally associated with motor control, is active in motor learning. The basal ganglia are also key elements in reward-based learning. Data from studies individuals with Tourette's syndrome, Obsessive-Compulsive Disorder as well as with Broca's aphasia, Parkinson's disease, hypoxia, focal brain damage, and from comparative studies of the brains and behavior of other species, demonstrate that the basal ganglia sequence the discrete elements that constitute a complete motor act, syntactic process, or thought process. Imaging studies of intact human subjects and electrophysiologic and tracer studies of the brains and behavior of other species confirm these findings. Dobzansky had stated, "Nothing in biology makes sense except in the light of evolution" (cited in [108]). That applies with as much force to the human brain and the neural bases of cognition as it does to the human foot or jaw. The converse follows: the mark of evolution on the brains of human beings and other species provides insight into the evolution of the brain bases of human language. The neural substrate that regulated motor control in the common ancestor of apes and humans most likely was modified to enhance cognitive and linguistic ability. Language and cognition played a central role in this process. However, the process that ultimately resulted in the human brain may have started when our earliest hominid ancestors began to walk.

Author details

Gerry Leisman
F.R. Carrick Institute for Clinical Ergonomics, Rehabilitation, and Applied Neurosciences, Garden City, New York USA
The National Institute for Brain and Rehabilitation Sciences, Nazareth, Israel
Nazareth Academic Institute, Nazareth, Israel
Biomedical Engineering, Dept. Biomechanics, ORT-Braude College of Engineering, Carmiel, Israel

Robert Melillo
F.R. Carrick Institute for Clinical Ergonomics, Rehabilitation, and Applied Neurosciences, Garden City, New York USA
The National Institute for Brain and Rehabilitation Sciences, Nazareth, Israel
Nazareth Academic Institute, Nazareth, Israel

Frederick R. Carrick
F.R. Carrick Institute for Clinical Ergonomics, Rehabilitation, and Applied Neurosciences, Garden City, New York USA
Carrick Institute for Graduate Studies, Cape Canaveral, Florida USA
Department of Neurology, Life University, Marietta, Georgia USA

Acknowledgement

This work was supported by the Ministry of Science of the State of Israel, the F., R. Carrick Research Institute, Inc., and Help the Hope Foundation.

11. References

[1] Thatch W.T Jr (1980). The Cerebellum, In: Mount Casgle D.D, editor, Medical Physiology, 14th edition. St. Louis, MO: Mosby, 837-858.
[2] Alexander G. E, Delong M.R, Strick P.L (1986) Parallel Organization of Functionally Segregated Circuits Linking Basal Ganglia and Cortex. Annu. rev. neurosci. 9:357-381.
[3] Alexander G.E, Crutcher M.D, Delong M.R (1990) Basal Ganglia–Thalamocortical Circuits: Parallel Substrates for Motor, Oculomotor, (Prefrontal) and (Limbic) Functions. In: Uylungs H.B.N, Van Eben C.G, DeBruin J.P.C, Corner M.A, Feenstra M.G.P editors. The Prefrontal Cortex, its Structure, Function, and Pathology. Amsterdam, the Netherlands: Elsevier, 266-271.
[4] Graybiel A.M (1995) Building action repertoires: memory and learning functions of the basal ganglia. Curr Opin Neurobiol.5(6):733-741.
[5] Féger J (1997) Updating the Functional Model of the Basal Ganglia. Trends neurosci. 20(4):152-153.
[6] Middleton, F.A, Strick P.L (2000) Basal Ganglia and Cerebellar Loops: Motor and Cognitive Circuits. Brain res rev. 31:236–250.
[7] Chudler E.H, Dong W.K (1995) The Role of the Bsal Ganglia in Nociception and Pain. Pain. 60(1):3-38.
[8] Middleton F.A, Strick P.L (1994) Anatomical Evidence for Cerebellar and Basal Ganglia Involvement in Higher Cognitive Function. Science. 266:458-461.
[9] Vitek JL, Giroux (2000) Physiology of Hypokinetic and Hyperkinetic Movement Disorders: Model for Dyskinesia. Ann neurol. 4(Suppl 1):S131-S140.
[10] Litvan I, Paulsen J.S, Mega M.S, Cummings J.L (1998) Neuropsychiatric Assessment of Patients with Hyperkinetic and Hypokinetic Movement Disorders. Arch neuro. 55:1313-1319.
[11] Stinear CM, Coxon JP, Byblow WD (2009) Primary Motor Cortex and Movement Prevention: Where Stop meets Go. Neurosci bobehav rev. 33(5):662-673.
[12] Yakimovskii A.F, Varshavskaya V.M (2004) Neostriatal Glutamatergic System is Involved in the Pathogenesis of Picrotoxin-Induced Choreomyoclonic Hyperkinesis. Bull exp biol med. 138(6):533-536.

[13] Kim J.M, Lee J.Y, Kim HJ, Kim JS, Kim YK, Park SS, Kim SE, Jeon BS (2010) The Wide Clinical Spectrum and Nigrostriatal Dopaminergic Damage in Spinocerebellar Ataxia Type 6. J neurol neurosurg psychiatry. 81(5):529-32.
[14] Lanska D.J (2010) The History of Movement Disorders. Handb clin neurol. 95:501-546.
[15] Cummings J.L, Diaz C, Levy M, Binetti G, Litvan I (1996) Neuropsychiatric Syndromes in Neurodegenerative Disease: Frequency and Signficance. Semin clin neuropsychiatry. 1(4):241-247.
[16] Litvan I, Mega M.S, Cummings J.L, Fairbanks L. (1996) Neuropsychiatric Aspects of Progressive Supranuclear Palsy. Neurol. 47(5):1184-1189.
[17] Fitzgerald K.D, Welsh R.C, Stern E.R, Angstadt M, Hanna G.L, Abelson J.L, Taylor S.F (2011) Developmental Alterations of Frontal-Striatal-Thalamic Connectivity in Obsessive-Compulsive Disorder. J am acad child adolesc psychiatry. 50(9):938-948.
[18] Gonçalves Ó.F, Carvalho S, Leite J, Pocinho F, Relvas J, Fregni F. (2011) Obsessive Compulsive Disorder as a Functional Interhemispheric Imbalance at the Thalamic Level. Med hypotheses. 77(3):445-447.
[19] van den Heuvel O.A, Mataix-Cols D, Zwitser G, Cath D.C, van der Werf Y.D, Groenewegen H.J, van Balkom A.J, Veltman D.J (2011) Common Limbic and Frontal-Striatal Disturbances in Patients with Obsessive Compulsive Disorder, Panic Disorder and Hypochondriasis. Psychol med. 41(11):2399-410.
[20] Chiu CH, Lo YC, Tang HS, Liu IC, Chiang WY, Yeh FC, Jaw FS, Tseng WY. (2011) White matter abnormalities of fronto-striato-thalamic circuitry in obsessive-compulsive disorder: A study using diffusion spectrum imaging tractography. Psychiatry Res. Jun 30;192(3):176-82.
[21] Wang Z, Maia T.V, Marsh R, Colibazzi T, Gerber A, Peterson B.S (2011) The Neural Circuits that Generate Tics in Tourette's Syndrome. Am j psychiatry. 168(12):1326-37.
[22] Du Y, Wu X, Li L (2011) Differentially Organized Top-Ddown Modulation of Prepulse Inhibition of Startle. J neurosci. 31(38):13644-13653.
[23] Jahfari S, Waldorp L, van den Wildenberg W.P, Scholte H.S, Ridderinkhof K.R, Forstmann B.U (2011) Effective Connectivity Reveals Important Roles for Both the Hyperdirect (Fronto-Subthalamic) and the Indirect (Fronto-Striatal-Pallidal) Fronto-Basal Ganglia Pathways During Response Inhibition. J neurosci. 31(18):6891-6899.
[24] Melillo R, Leisman G (2009a). Neurobehavioral Disorders of Childhood: An Evoloutionary Approach, New York, NY: Springer.
[25] Nambu A, Chiken S, Shashidharan P, Nishibayashi H, Ogura M, Kakishita K, Tanaka S, Tachibana Y, Kita H, Itakura T (2011) Reduced Pallidal Output Causes Dystonia. Front syst neurosci. 5:89.
[26] Vitek J.L, Zhang J, Hashimoto T, Russo G.S, Baker K.B (2012) External Pallidal Stimulation Improves Parkinsonian Motor Signs and Modulates Neuronal Activity Throughout the Basal Ganglia Thalamic Network. Exp neurol. 233(1):581-586.
[27] Mendoza J.E, Foundas A.F (2008) Clinical Neuroanatomy: A Neurobehavioral Approach, New York, NY: Springer, 2008, pp. 153-193.

[28] Kalva S.K, Rengaswamy M, Chakravarthy V.S, Gupte N (2012) On the Neural Substrates for Exploratory Dynamics in Basal Ganglia: A Model. Neural netw. 2012 Feb 14. [Epub ahead of print]

[29] Leisman G, Machado C, Melillo R, Mualem R (2012) Intentionality and 'Free-Will' From a Neurodevelopmental Perspective. Front integr neurosci. 2012 [In Press].

[30] Leisman G, Melillo R (2012) The Development of the Frontal Lobes in Infancy and Childhood: Asymmetry and the Nature of Temperament and Adjustment. In: Cavanna, A.E editor. Frontal Lobe: Anatomy, Functions and Injuries. Hauppauge, NY: Nova Scientific Publishers.

[31] Leisman G (1976) The Role of Visual Processes in Attention and its Disorders. In: Leisman G editor Basic Visual Processes and Learning Disability. Springfield, Il: Charles C. Thomas, 7-123.

[32] Ridding M.C, Sheean G, Rothwell J.C, Inzelberg R, Kujirai T (1995) Changes in the Balance Between Motor Cortical Excitation and Inhibition in Focal, Task Specific Dystonia. J neurol neurosurg psychiatry. 59(5):493-8.

[33] Wolosin S.M, Richardson M.E, Hennessey J.G, Denckla M.B, Mostofsky S.H (2009) Abnormal Cerebral Cortex Structure in Children with ADHD. Hum brain mapp. 30(1):175-184.

[34] Lee J.S, Kim B.N, Kang E, Lee D.S, Kim Y.K, Chung J.K, Lee M.C, Cho S.C (2005) Regional Cerebral Blood Flow in Children with Attention Deficit Hyperactivity Disorder: Comparison Before and After Methylphenidate Treatment. Hum brain mapp. 24(3):157-164.

[35] Kang D-H, Davidson R.J, Coe C.L, Wheeler R.E, Tomarken A.J, Ershler W.B (1991) Frontal Brain Asymmetry and Immune Function. Behav neurosci. 105(6):860-869.

[36] Bal T, Debay D, Destexhe A (2000) Cortical Feedback Controls the Frequency and Synchrony of Oscillations in the Visual Thalamus. J neurosci. 20(19):7478–7488.

[37] Aron AR, Poldrack RA (2006). Cortical and subcortical contributions to Stop signal response inhibition: role of the subthalamic nucleus. J neurosci. 26(9):2424-2433.

[38] Schmahmann JD, Pandya DN. (2008). Disconnection Syndromes of Basal Ganglia, Thalamus, and Cerebrocerebellar Systems. Cortex. 44(8):1037-1066.

[39] Blood AJ. (2008) New Hypotheses About Postural Control Support The Notion that all Dystonias are Manifestations of Excessive Brain Postural Function. Biosci Hypotheses. 1(1):14-25.

[40] Marsden CD, Rothwell JC. (1987). The Physiology of Idiopathic Dystonia. Can J Neurol Sci. 14(3 Suppl):521-527.

[41] Mitra S, Knight A, Munn A. (2012). Divergent Effects of Cognitive Load on Quiet Stance and Task-Linked Postural Coordination. J Exp Psychol Hum Percept Perform. Nov 5. [Epub ahead of print]

[42] Fujiwara K, Yaguchi C, Kunita K, Mammadova A. (2012) Effects of neck flexion on discriminative and cognitive processing in anticipatory postural control during bilateral arm movement. Neurosci Lett. 518(2):144-148.

[43] Litvan I, Mohr E, Williams J, Gomez C, Chase T.N (1991) Differential memory and executive functions in demented patients with Parkinson's and Alzheimer's disease. J neurol. neurosurg psychiat. 54(1):25-29.

[44] Zeef D.H, Vlamings R, Lim L.W, Tan S, Janssen M.L, Jahanshahi A, Hoogland G, Prickaerts J, Steinbusch H.W, Temel Y (2012) Motor and Non-motor Behaviour in Experimental Huntington's Disease. Behav brain res. 226(2):435-439.

[45] Cummings J.L, Cunningham K. (1992) Obsessive-Compulsive Disorder in Huntington's Disease. Biol psychiatry. 31(3):263-270.

[46] Cummings J.L (1993) Frontal-Subcortical Circuits and Human Behavior. Arch neurol. 50(8):873-880.

[47] Coffey B.J, Miguel E.C, Biederman J, Baer L, Rauch S.L, O'Sullivan R.L, Savage C.R, Phillips K, Borgman A, Green-Leibovitz M.I, Moore E, Park K.S, Jenike M.A (1998) Tourette's Disorder with and without Obsessive-Compulsive Disorder in Adults: Are they Different? J nerv ment dis. 186(4):201-6.

[48] Beaulieu J.M, Gainetdinov R.R (2011) The Physiology, Signaling, and Pharmacology of Dopamine Receptors. Pharmacol rev. 63(1):182-217.

[49] Sturrock A, Laule C, Decolongon J, Dar Santos R, Coleman A.J, Creighton S, Bechtel N, Reilmann R, Hayden M.R, Tabrizi S.J, Mackay A.L, Leavitt B.R. (2010) Magnetic Resonance Spectroscopy Biomarkers in Premanifest and Early Huntington Disease. Neurology. 75(19):1702-1710.

[50] Grahn J.A, Parkinson J.A, Owen A.M. (2009) The Role of the Basal Ganglia in Learning and Memory: Neuropsychological Studies. Behav brain res. 199(1):53-60.

[51] Gomez-Tortosa E, Arias-Navalon J.A, Barrio-Alba A, Barroso F.T, Pardo Pardo C, Sánchez Martín J.A, García Yébenes J (1996) Relation Between Frontal Lobe Blood Flow and Cognitive Performance in Huntington's Disease. Neurologia. 11, 251-256.

[52] Weinberger D.R, Berman K.F, Ladarola N, Driesen N, Zec R.F (1988) Free Frontal Cortical Blood Flow and Cognitive Function in Huntington's Disease. J neurol neurosurg psychiatry. 51, 94-104.

[53] Brooks D.J, Turjanski N, Sawle G.V, Playford E.D, Lees A.J (1992) PET Studies of the Integrity of the Pre and Postsynaptic Dopaminergic System in Tourette Syndrome. Adv neurol. 58:227–231.

[54] Brooks D.J (1993) PET Studies on the Early and Differential Diagnosis of Parkinson's Disease. Neurology. 43(12 Suppl 6):S6-S16.

[55] Tamm L, Menon V, Ringel J, Reiss A.L (2004) Event-Related fMRI Evidence of Frontotemporal Involvement in Aberrant Response Inhibition and Task Switching in Attention-Deficit/Hyperactivity Disorder. J am acad child adolesc psychiatry. 43(11):1430-1440.

[56] Bush G, Valera E.M, Seidman L.J (2005) Functional Neuroimaging of Attention-Deficit/Hyperactivity Disorder: A review and Suggested Future Directions Biol psychiatry. 57:1273–1284.

[57] Zarei M, Mataix-Cols D, Heyman I, Hough M, Doherty J, Burge L, Winmill L, Nijhawan S, Matthews P.M, James A (2011) Changes in Gray Matter Volume and White Matter

Microstructure in Adolescents with Obsessive-Compulsive Disorder. Biol psychiatry. 70(11):1083-1090.

[58] Harrison B.J, Soriano-Mas C, Pujol J, Ortiz H, López-Solà M, Hernández-Ribas R, Deus J, Alonso P, Yücel M, Pantelis C, Menchon J.M, Cardoner N. (2009) Altered Corticostriatal Functional Connectivity in Obsessive-Compulsive dDsorder. Arch gen psychiatry. 66(11):1189-1200.

[59] Maia T.V, Cooney R.E, Peterson B.S (2008) The neural bases of Obsessive-Compulsive Disorder in Children and Adults. Dev psychopathol. 20(4):1251-1283.

[60] Schwartz J.M, Stoessel P.W, Baxter Jr. L.R, , Martin K.M, Phelps M.E (1996) Systematic Changes in Cerebral Glucose Metabolic Rate after Successful Behaviour Modification Treatment of Obsessive Compulsive Disorder. Arch gen psychiatry. 53:109–113.

[61] Adams K.H, Hansen E.S, Pinborg L.H, Hasselbalch S.G, Svarer C, Holm S, Bolwig T.G, Knudsen G.M (2005) Patients with Obsessive-Compulsive Disorder have Increased 5-HT2A Receptor Binding in the Caudate Nuclei. Int j neuropsychopharmacol. 8(3):391-401.

[62] Ho Pian K.L, van Megen H.J, Ramsey N.F, Mandl R, van Rijk P.P, Wynne H.J, Westenberg H.G (2005) Decreased Thalamic Blood Flow in Obsessive-Compulsive Disorder Patients Responding to Fluvoxamine. Psychiatry res. 138(2):89-97.

[63] Sears L.L, Vest C, Mohamed S, Bailey J, Ranson B.J, Piven J (1999) An MRI Study of the Basal Ganglia in Autism. Prog neuropsychopharmacol biol psychiatry. 23:613–624.

[64] Melillo R, Leisman G (2009) Autism Spectrum Disorder as Functional Disconnection Syndrome. Rev neurosci. 20:2,111-132.

[65] Nordahl C.W, Lange N, Li D.D, Barnett L.A, Lee A, Buonocore M.H, Simon T.J, Rogers S, Ozonoff S, Amaral D.G (2011) Brain Enlargement is Associated with Regression in Preschool-Age Boys with Autism Spectrum Disorders. Proc natl acad sci USA. 108(50):20195-20200.

[66] Howe M.W, Atallah H.E, McCool A, Gibson D.J, Graybiel A.M (2011) Habit Learning is Associated with Major Shifts in Frequencies of Oscillatory Activity and Synchronized Spike Firing in Striatum. Proc natl acad sci USA. 108(40):16801-16806.

[67] Lingawi N.W, Balleine B.W (2012) Amygdala Central Nucleus Interacts with Dorsolateral Striatum to Regulate the Acquisition of Habits. J neurosci. 32(3):1073-1081.

[68] Graybiel A.M, Rauch S.L (2000) Toward a neurobiology of Obsessive-Compulsive Disorder. Neuron. 28:343–347.

[69] Tobe R.H, Bansal R, Xu D, Hao X, Liu J, Sanchez J, Peterson B.S (2010) Cerebellar Morphology in Tourette Syndrome and Obsessive-Compulsive Disorder. Ann neurol. 67(4):479-487.

[70] Marsh R, Maia T.V, Peterson B.S (2009) Functional Disturbances within Frontostriatal Circuits Across Multiple Childhood Psychopathologies. Am j psychiatry. 166(6):664-74.

[71] Amat J.A, Bronen R.A, Saluja S, Sato N, Zhu H, Gorman D.A, Royal J Peterson BS. (2006) Increased Number of Subcortical Hyperintensities on MRI in Children and Adolescents with Tourette's Syndrome, Obsessive-Compulsive Disorder, and Attention Deficit Hyperactivity Disorder. Am j psychiatry. 163(6):1106-1108.

[72] Canales J.J, Graybiel A.M (2000) A Measure of Striatal Function Predicts Motor Stereotypy. Nat neurosci. 3(4):377-383.

[73] Fan Q, Tan L, You C, Wang J, Ross C.A, Wang X, Zhang T, Li J, Chen K, Xiao Z (2010) Increased N-Acetylaspartate/creatine Ratio ithe Medial Prefrontal Cortex Among Unmedicated Obsessive-Compulsive Disorder Patients. Psychiatry clin neurosci. 64(5):483-490.

[74] Matsunaga H, Hayashida K, Maebayashi K, Mito H, Kiriike N (2011) A Case Series of Aripiprazole Augmentation of Selective Serotonin Reuptake Inhibitors in Treatment-Refractory Obsessive Compulsive Disorder. Int j psychiatry clin pract. 15(4):263-269.

[75] el Mansari M, Bouchard C, Blier P (1995) Alteration of Serotonin Release in the Guinea Pig Orbito-Frontal Cortex by Selective Serotonin Reuptake Inhibitors. Relevance to Treatment of Obsessive-Compulsive Disorder. Neuropsychopharmacol. 13(2):117-127.

[76] Leckman J, Cohen D (1999) Tourette's Syndrome – Tics, Obsessions, Compulsions: Developmental Psychopathology and Clinical Care. New York: Wiley.

[77] Peterson B, Leckman J.F (1998) A Functional Magnetic Resonance Imaging Study of Tic Suppression in Tourette Syndrome. Arch gen psychiatry 55, 326–333.

[78] Cavanna A.E, Termine C (2012) Tourette Syndrome. Adv exp med biol. 724:375-383.

[79] Mink J.W (2001) Basal Ganglia Dysfunction in Tourette's Syndrome: A New Hypothesis. Pediatr neurol. 25:190–198.

[80] Pulst S.M, Walshe T.M, Romero J.A (1983) Carbon Monoxide Poisoning with Features of Gilles de la Tourette's Syndrome Arch Neurol. 40(7):443-444.

[81] Pringsheim T, Doja A, Gorman D, McKinlay D, Day L, Billinghurst L, Carroll A, Dion Y, Luscombe S, Steeves T, Sandor P. (2012) Canadian Guidelines for the Evidence-Based Treatment of Tic Disorders: Pharmacotherapy. Can j psychiatry. 57(3):133-143.

[82] Gurevich E.V, Joyce J.N (1996) Comparison of [3H]paroxetine and [3H]cyanoimipramine for Quantitative Measurement of Serotonin Transporter Sites in Human Brain. Neuropsychopharmacol. 14, 309–323.

[83] Van Bockstaele E.J, Cestari D.M, Pickel V.M (1994) Synaptic Structure and Connectivity of Serotonin Terminals in the Ventral Tegmental Area: Potential Sites for Modulation of Mesolimbic Dopamine Neurons. Brain res. 647, 307–322.

[84] Lambe E.K, Krimer L.S, Goldman-Rakic P.S (2000) Differential Postnatal Development of Catecholamine and Serotonin Inputs to Identified Neurons in Prefrontal Cortex of Rhesus Monkey. J neurosci. 20:8780–8787.

[85] Bolam, J.P., Hanley JJ, Booth PA, Bevan MD. (2000) Synaptic Organisation of the Basal Ganglia. J anat. 196:527–542.

[86] Kelly A.E, Berridge K.C (2002) The Neuroscience of Natural Rewards: Relevance to Addictive Drugs. J neurosci. 22:3306–3311.

[87] Nicola S.M, Surmeier J, Malenka R.C (2000) Dopaminergic Modulation of Neuronal Excitability in the Striatum and Nucleus Accumbens. Annu rev. Neurosci. 23:185–215.

[88] Darwin C. (1998) *The Expression of the Emotions in Man and Animals.* In: Ekman P, editor New York: Oxford.

[89] Packard M.G, Knowlton B (2002) Learning and Memory Functions of the Basal Ganglia. Annu. rev Neurosci. 25:563–593.

[90] Seymour B, O'Doherty J.P, Dayan P, Koltzenburg M, Jones A.K, Dolan R.J, Friston K.J, Frackowiak R.S. (2004) Temporal Difference Models Describe Higher-Order Learning in Humans. Nature. 429(6992):664-667.

[91] Minamimoto T, Hori Y, Kimura M (2005) Complementary Process to Response Bias in the Centromedian Nucleus of the Thalamus. Science 308:1798–1801.

[92] Mink J.W (1996) The Basal Ganglia: Focused Selection and Inhibition of Competing Motor Programs. Prog Neurobiol. 50:381–425.

[93] Albin R.L, Mink J.W (2006) Recent Advances in Tourette Syndrome Research. Trends Neurosci. 29:3:175-182.

[94] Teicher M.H, Anderson C.M, Polcari A, Glod C.A, Maas L.C, Renshaw P.F. (2000) Functional Deficits In Basal Ganglia of Children with Attention-Deficit/Hyperactivity Disorder Shown with Functional Magnetic Resonance Imaging Relaxometry. Nat Med. 6(4):470-473.

[95] Castellanos F.X, Lee P.P, Sharp W, Jeffries N.O, Greenstein D.K, Clasen L.S, Blumenthal J.D, James R.S, Ebens C.L, Walter J.M, Zijdenbos A, Evans A.C, Giedd J.N, Rapoport J.L (2002) Developmental Trajectories of Brain Volume Abnormalities in Children and Adolescents with Attention-Deficit/Hyperactivity Disorder. JAMA. 288(14):1740-1748.

[96] Sergeant J.A, Geurts H, Oosterlaan J (2002) How Specific is a Deficit of Executive Functioning for Attention-Deficit/Hyperactivity Disorder? Behav brain res. 130:3–28.

[97] Semrud-Clikeman M, Steingard RJ, Filipek P, Biederman J, Bekken K, Renshaw PF (2000) Using MRI to Examine Brain-Behavior Relationships in Males with Attention Deficit Disorder with Hyperactivity. J am acad child adolesc psychiatry. 39(4):477-84.

[98] Bush G, Frazier J.A, Rauch S.L, Seidman L.J, Whalen P.J, Jenike M.A, Rosen B.R, Biederman J (1999) Anterior Cingulate Cortex Dysfunction in Attention-Deficit/Hyperactivity Disorder Revealed by FMRI and the Counting Stroop. Biol psychiatry 45:1542–1552.

[99] Vaidya C.J, Austin G, Kirkorian G, Ridlehuber H.W, Desmond J.E, Glover G.H, Gabrielli J.D (1998) Selective Effects of Methylphenidate in Attention Deficit Hyperactivity Disorder: A Functional Magnetic Resonance Study. Proc natl acad sci USA. 95:14494–14499.

[100] Durston S, Thomas K.M, Worden M.S, Yang Y, Casey B.J (2002) The Effect of Preceding Context on Inhibition: An Event-Related FMRI Study. Neuroimage. 16(2):449-453.

[101] Qiu A, Crocetti D, Adler M, Mahone E.M, Denckla M.B, Miller M.I, Mostofsky S.H, (2009) Basal Ganglia Volume and Shape in Children With Attention Deficit Hyperactivity Disorder. Am j psychiatry. 166(1): 74–82.

[102] Aron, A.R, Durston S, Eagle D.M, Logan G.D, Stinear C.M, Stuphorn V (2007) Converging Evidence for a Fronto-Basal-Ganglia Network for Inhibitory Control of Action and Cognition. J neurosci. 27(44):11860 –11864.

[103] Aron A.R, Fletcher P.C, Bullmore E.T, Sahakian B.J, Robbins T.W (2003). Stop Signal Inhibition Disrupted by Damage to Right Inferior Frontal Gyrus in Humans. Nat neurosci. 6:115–116.

[104] Chambers C.D, Bellgrove M.A, Stokes M.G, Henderson T.R, Garavan H, Robertson I.H, Morris A.P, Mattingley J.B (2006) Executive "Brake Failure" Following Deactivation of Human Frontal Lobe. J Cogn Neurosci. 18:444–455.

[105] Aron A.R, Poldrack R.A (2006) Cortical and Subcortical Contributions to Stop Signal Response Inhibition: Role of The Subthalamic Nucleus. J neurosci. 26:2424 –2433.

[106] Floden D, Stuss D.T (2006) Inhibitory Control is Slowed in Patients with Right Superior Medial Frontal Damage. J cogn neurosci. 18:1843–1849.

[107] Nachev P, Wydell H, O'Neill K, Husain M, Kennard C (2007) The Role of The Pre-Supplementary Motor Area in the Control of Action. NeuroImage. 36 [Suppl 2]:T155–T163.

[108] Mayr E (1982) The Growth of Biological Thought. Diversity, Evolution, and Inheritance. Cambridge, Mass.: Harvard University Press.

Chapter 2

Fetal and Environmental Basis for the Cause of Parkinson's Disease

Clivel G. Charlton

Additional information is available at the end of the chapter

http://dx.doi.org/10.5772/52680

1. Introduction

In Parkinson's disease (PD) dopamine producing neurons in the substantia nigra, pars compacta of the midbrain and with their axons projecting to the neostriatum degenerate. PD is classified as being familiar when it is known to be the result of genetic abnormalities, and this represents about 5 to 10 percent of all cases. The other cases are idiopathic, represent 90 – 95 percent of all cases of PD and the causes are unknown. The expression of the specific symptoms of idiopathic PD vary among individuals, and may be accompanied with other brain disorders, including Alzheimer's type dementia, depression and amyotrophic lateral sclerosis (ALS). The common relationship among all of the degenerative disorders is that all are caused by failure of specific functions that are under the control of identifiable neuronal sets, with relatively low population number of larger neurons that usually occur in clusters and with far reaching axons. These neurons are well represented by the nigrostriatal dopamine neurons, and the degeneration of the neuronal set represents the major pathology of PD. They are also represented by the basal nucleus of Meynert acetylcholine neurons with major projections to the cerebral cortex that degenerate in Alzheimer's disease (AD), and by the upper and lower motor neurons with projections to the brainstem, spinal cord or motor-end plate, that degenerate in ALS. These neuronal sets have specific prenatal and fetal periods for their neurogenesis, migration and axonal extension during which they acquire their specific phenotype that can be influenced by internally and externally derived biochemical forces, including toxins and excesses and deficiency of regulatory factors that will shape the physiological and functional destiny of these neuronal sets. If the influence is of a positive or enhancing nature, the neuronal set will turn out to be functionally superior or with exceptional resilience and longevity and will impart an enhanced character to the individual. However, if the influence is deleterious it will cause harm to the neuronal set and likewise will influence the character of the individual. For the latter, deficiencies may occur at sub-threshold level, may continue in a subliminal and a graded way and may compromise resilience and functional longevity, finally serving as the 'weak link' and pairing with deteriorating changes that occur during aging to cause diseases, such as Parkinson's disease. Whereas the gene has inherent command over the variation of biological forms and some biological outcomes, it is the interacting entities derived from the environment that really sway functional outcomes. Toxins, that may be endogenous or exogenous, represent a set of these environmental factors and quite likely are responsible for the cause of idiopathic PD and other degenerative disorders. So, this chapter will discuss the idea, supported by experimental findings, that the substantia nigra dopamine neurons that deteriorate to the point of causing idiopathic PD were impaired early in life at a sub-threshold level. This occurs during the vulnerable stage of neurogenesis, neuronal development and neuronal migration. The exposures of the substantia nigra dopamine neurons to toxic or harmful influences early in life cause sub-threshold harm, and further exposures to stress during aging cause additive insults that precipitate the symptoms of PD. The early insults, the naturally low population of nigrostriatal neurons, the continuous functional demands placed on the few nigrostriatal DA neurons and the far-reaching nature of the axonal projections render the nigrostriatal DA neurons vulnerable. The high content of cytoskeleton and their kinases seen as pathological markers for various degenerative disorders (McGee and Steele, 2011) indicate that axonal damage to far-reaching neurons is a preeminent occurrence in PD.

2. Major symptoms and the proposed causes for Parkinson's disease

The major clinical symptoms of Parkinson's disease (PD), an age-related disorder, are resting tremors, hypokinesia, rigidity and postural instability (Tetriakoff, 1919: Foix and Nicolesco, 1925) caused by the degeneration of the nigrostriatal (NS) dopaminergic pathway and the depletion of dopamine (DA) (Greenfield and Bosanquet, 1953; Hornykiewicz, 1966). The pathological features include extensive (about 70% or more) loss of dopaminergic neurons in the pars compacta of the substantia nigra, the presence of inter-cytoplasmic inclusions known as Lewy's bodies and gliosis. It was reported also that norepinephrine (NE) (Erhinger and Hornykiewicz, 1960) and serotonin (5-HT) Bernheimer et al., 1961) levels are decreased and that acetylcholine neurotransmission (Yahr, 1968) is increased. A small population of PD cases is caused by genetic abnormalities, involving alpha–synuclein (Polymeropoulos et al, 1997; Papadimitrior et al, 1999 and Kruger et al,1998, Dauer et al, 2002), ubiquitin (Leroy et al, 1998) and apolipoprotein E (APOE), (Kruger et al, 1999). Changes in chromosome 2p13 (Gasser et al, 1998), cyp2D6 (Kruger et al, 1999; Christensen et al, 1998; Kosel et al, 1996; Bon et al, 1999, Sabbagh et al, 1999) as well as mitochondria tRNA (A4336G) (Epensperger et al, 1997) have also been reported. The mutation of the parkin gene is closely associated with juvenile PD (Kitada et al, 1998), which has about eight variants (Lansbury and Brice, 2002). It should be noted however, that multiple other PD cases have been screened and they did not harbor mutations (Giasson et al, 2000), but gene mutations may serve as vulnerable markers, superimposed by environmental factors and age-related wear-and–tear. The root-cause of idiopathic PD is unknown, but various factors are implicated, including the oxidation of dopamine, free radical-mediated oxidative injury, mitochondrial abnormalities, excitotoxins, over exposure to manganese (Chu et al, 1995; Hochberg et al, 1996) and carbon monoxide, the intake of beta-methylaminoalanine (Spencer, 1987), benzyl-tetra-hydroisoquinolines and tetra-hydroprotoberines (Caparros-Lefebvre and Steele, 2005), 1-methyl-4-phenyl-1,2,3,6-tetrahydropyridine (Davis et al, 1979), methanol (Guggenheim et al, 1971). As well as the potent methylating agent, methylazoxymethanol (Ince and Codd, 2005) and excess methylation via high utilization of the endogenous S-adenosyl-L- methionine in the brain (Charlton and Way, 1978; Charlton et al, 1992; Charlton and Mack, 1994).

2.1. Aberrations in non-basal ganglia systems

In PD the basal ganglia is the primary affected structure, but lesions have been identified in the locus ceruleus (Selby, 1968; Alvord et al, 1974), the hypothalamus (Jagar and Bethlem, 1969; Ohama and Ikuta, 1976; Langston and Forno, 1978), the dorsal motor nucleus of vagus (Eadie, 1963; Vanderhaegen et al 1970), the sympathetic ganglia (Jagar and Bethlem, 1960; Vanderhaeghen et al., 1970; Rajput and Rozdilsky, 1970 and Forno and Norvill, 1976) and in the adrenal medulla (Jager, 1969) as well. Furthermore, Lewy's bodies, the standard marker for PD, have been seen in the cerebral cortex, anterior thalamus, hypothalamus, amygdala, basal forebrain, dorsal motor nucleus of vagus, adrenal medulla and locus ceruleus. The clearly un-circumscribed localization of lesions in the patients or victims of PD means that the changes or the incidents that cause the dopaminergic cell loss in the nigrostriatal system may not specifically target the basal ganglia, but instead the nigrostriatal dopaminergic neurons may be more vulnerable or sensitive. In other words, the factors that are involved in the cause of, at least, some cases of PD may also cause harm to other cell populations, but the basal ganglia neurons are more vulnerable and will die when other neuronal sets remain alive and function normally. This means that a state of vulnerability or sensitization may exists for PD and that the occurrence of damage to other neuronal pool may help to explain the variation in the expression of the PD syndrome.

3. The fetal basis hypothesis for Parkinson's disease

PD is age-related but a large percentage of the older population does not suffer from the disorder, although aging is accompanied with pronounced and progressing reduction in motor and other functions. The age-dependent increase in the frequency of essential tremor (Elble 1995; Koller and Huber, 1989), the occurrence of kyphotic posture, diminished arm swing, shorter strides (Murray et al, 1969; Elble et al, 1992; Elble et al, 1991, bradykinesia (Waite et al, 1996) and slowed reaction time (Weiss 1965; Welford, 1977) are signs found to be associated with aging, but the abnormalities are distinguishable from the changes that occur in PD. This suggests that, during normal aging and as a rule, the nigrostriatal DA neurons do not deteriorate to the point of causing PD. Therefore, it is very possible that for PD symptoms to be expressed in the aged, some primary changes that render the nigrostriatal DA neurons vulnerable occur during the earlier life of the PD patients and serve as the underpinning for the deleterious age-related changes that normally occur. So, the functional age-related changes pair with the early predispositions to precipitate the symptoms of PD. Furthermore, there is the high probability that the causes of the vulnerability that occur early in life are based on chance and occur during a critical period when nigrostriatal dopamine neurons are structurally responsive to endogenous and exogenous toxic type of interventions.

3.1. Chance encounter of the nigrostriatal neurons with harmful factors

It is proposed that chance encounter of factors with the NS DA neurons at critical times during their development eventually shape the long-term outcome of the neuronal pool. If the encounter decreases the longevity of the neurons idiopathic PD will occur. This will underlie the sporadic feature of idiopathic PD, and the nature of the early encounter will determine the pathological characteristics. So, the cluster of PD cases caused by the outbreak of the epidemic encephalitis lethargic in 1919 that killed about one million people worldwide and left millions more 'frozen' with the symptoms of PD and which decline rapidly after 1925 (Ravenholt et al, 1982) represent a special but a typical set of parkinsonism. The Guam Parkinson's dementia complex (PDC)-amyotrophic lateral sclerosis (ALS) syndrome proposed to be caused by the toxins contained in flour prepared from the cycad plant (Spencer et al, 1987) suggests a syndrome that is caused by long–term exposures that target the nigrostriatal neurons, motor neurons and basal nucleus of Meynert acetlycholinergic neurons. In these cases the diversity in the character of the syndrome is a reflection of the neuronal sets that were harmed. So, the individuals that develop idiopathic Parkinson's disease, and likely other neurodegenerative disorders, were marked early in life for the disorder. The early process may be synonymous to natural selection that occurs by chance, and helps to define the variation of phenotypes among a population. In the case of PD, the variation may be defined by the magnitude of the reduction in the number of nigrostriatal dopaminergic neurons, and/or deficiencies in the metabolic capability or resilience of the neurons. Therefore, the nigrostriatal DA neurons of the PD patients may have experienced early exposure to environmental, nutritional and/or metabolic toxic interventions. This early exposures may result in DA neurons that lack the reserve capacity to survive during the natural life of the individual, but they function at a level of output that is above the threshold at which the symptoms of PD occur (pre-threshold). During the progression of time or during aging, however, subtle but accumulative changes occur that further damage the nigrostriatal DA neurons and the additive effects precipitate PD-like symptoms. **Thus, the fetal basis hypothesis proposes that by chance early interventions render the nigrostriatal neurons sensitive, susceptible or vulnerable, characteristics that enable changes involving the wear-and-tear of living or the exposure to toxins or traumatic events later in life to take a toll on the vulnerable NS neurons and cause PD.**

3.2. High workload may explain the vulnerability of the nigrostriatal neurons

The normal population of nigrostriatal pigmented neurons is relatively low, showing a mean value of 163,238 ± 42,372 in normal human (Ma et al, 1997). The relatively low population number of the nigrostriatal neurons and the high workload placed on these specialized cells play a role in their metabolic durability. This relationship may help to explain the rapid decline in the ability to effectively execute rapid and skillful movement-related skills as a function of aging. This is evident in the short time that a competitive athlete can maintain his or her exceptional ability. A 100-meter runner, for example, is normally competitive for only one or two olympic game and skillful ballet dancers are young people. Even the ability to play the game of golf requires skills that deteriorate to non-competitiveness by the time the athlete reaches early middle age. So, even under normal living condition the nigrostriatal neurons are under moment-by-moment demands by the motor and other functions that they control, and their capability naturally deteriorates in time. The demands placed on these neurons by muscles, for example, are continuously occurring, even during sleep, since skeletal muscle activities are maintained for limb and eye movements. Demands on the nigrostriatal neurons are continuous during regular activities and increased during stress-related physical activities, so, these neurons never rest, unlike neurons that control functions such as hearing, vision and cognition that are at rest at least during sleep. Therefore, while other neuronal sets with less stressful functions and without experiencing an early assault will age at a regular rate, the functional stress imposed on already susceptible dopamine neurons, during the process of living, will cause them to deteriorate at a fast rate to below the threshold that maintains normal functions. This means, therefore, that the prenatal exposure hypothesis will explain cases of juvenile PD that occur at about the age of forty years, in patients that are functionally normal high into the thirties. So, early markers for juvenile PD that are known to be caused by genetic abnormalities, likely exist long before the occurrence of the PD symptoms. The early markers may exist as subtle but serious sub-threshold genetic nigrostriatal abnormality that is below the threshold at which PD symptoms are expressed. So, as compared to idiopathic PD, that has its onset about in the sixth decade, juvenile PD, because of it more serious early impairments, requires a shorter duration of time before the added stress induces threshold level nigrostriatal damage. The overall analogy, therefore, means that at least two stages or two sets of factors or groups of factors are involved in PD:

1. The first stage: the predisposing/sensitization/susceptible/vulnerable stage.
2. The second stage: the inducing/precipitating/superimposing stage.

Again, the first stage is defined by subtle or sub-threshold level of adverse changes that start early in life and form the weak link for the second stage, defined by stressful events occurring later in life and coupled with the first stage to cause the expression of the disease symptoms. It should be noted that normal functional and age-related existence may cause enough stress to produce the 'added-on' second stage damage to the nigrostriatal neurons in individuals with early stage predisposition.

4. The predisposing, sensitization, susceptible or vulnerable stage of the hypothesis

Normally, immature neurons or neuroblast are subject to chemical and mechanical influences that cause them to migrate to various locations in the nervous system, to extend axonal and dendritic processes toward other cells and then to make and break synaptic connections with these cells before a final pattern of branching and connections are established (Levitan and Kaczmarek, 2002). Moreover, factors released by other cells influence the type of neurotransmitter the neuron will synthesize and the specific type and mixture of receptor, ion channels and other proteins that determine the characteristics of the fully differentiated neurons (Levitan and Kaczmarek, 2002). Along with or besides the normal pattern of development that occur, the differentiating and young neurons may be subjected to toxic and interfering influences that shape them for life. There could be failure in the normal process of apoptosis, that acts via cytochrome c, caspase 9, caspase 3 and other cellular constituents, to cause cellular pruning and to allow the remaining neurons to survive and to be properly organized.

In general, brain neurons are known to be susceptible or vulnerable to insults during prenatal and the early postnatal stage of the life of the individual. This is the basic reasons for the practice of protecting the pregnant mother, new born and young children from chemical and other potentially harmful exposures. For the midbrain dopaminergic system, the most susceptible time is likely to be the period of neurogenesis, proliferation and migration of the cells to produce the nigrostriatal dopaminergic phenotype. These midbrain dopamine neurons are generated early during development, first in the midbrain-hindbrain junction (Voorn et al, 1988), and they migrated radially to their final position in the ventral midbrain to form the substantia nigra, the ventral tegmental area and the retrorubal nuclei (Perrone-Capano and di Porzio 1996). Tyrosine hydroxylase (TH) immunoreactivity is used to identify those dopamine tegmental neurons, and the first appearance of the TH marker is regarded as the birth of the tegmental cells, which occurs on embryonic day 9 for the mouse. The periods close to the birth of these neurons are likely to be a very critical window through which the environment causes long-term changes to the cells and to the motor performance of the organism. In fact, it is these types of manipulations that may be relevant in causing diseases and in enhancing special features related to the functions of the basal ganglia, and they will have effects similar to natural selection and imprinting.

The signal for the differentiation of the NS DA neurons is through a protein called the sonic hedgehog (SHH). The amino-terminal product is the inductive moiety. SHH is produced by the floor plate cells and induces the dopaminergic phenotype (Hayes, et al., 1995). The signal for the SHH protein can be antagonized by increasing the activity of cyclic AMP-dependent protein kinase A. High activity of cAMP blocked the induction of dopamine neurons (Hayes et al, 1995), therefore it could be reasoned that other molecules, e.g. environmental toxins, that modulate cyclic AMP-dependent protein kinase A will interfere with cellular differentiation and migration of these emerging DA neurons. Biomolecules may also affect the metabolic and structural components of the emerging DA neurons, resulting in different degrees of effects that may be enhancing or detrimental to the functions and longevity of the new born DA neurons. If the modulation enhances the metabolism and functions of the nigrostriatal neurons it is expected that the adult may possess motor features that are superior in functions, and will endure to advance ages. On the other hand if the modulations impair metabolism and functions of the nigrostriatal neurons, it is expected that the adult will possess motor features that fail early in life to produce PD symptoms. So, the severity of the prenatal impairment will dictate the age of onset of PD symptoms. Susceptible type of impairments that are most severe, and do not result in death of the fetus, will be closest to the threshold at which PD symptoms are seen, so patients with early onset or juvenile PD may be endowed with sub-threshold but severely impaired NS system that developed early in life.

In summary, the period for the reorganization of the cellular membranes, organization of the chromatid for cell division, the synthesis of structural proteins, production of sub-systems for neurotransmitter synthesis and storage and the synthesis of molecules for intracellular transport and cell movement make the emerging dopaminergic cells well exposed to interfering factors and incidents. During this transforming cellular period the lack of essential metabolites, exposure to inappropriate metabolites and to exogenous and/or endogenous toxins can interfere with the molecular processes to cause permanent changes to the differentiating and migrating cells, that will reduce the resilience of the cell population. The affected neuronal set will become sensitive, susceptible, predisposed or vulnerable to the "wear-and-tear" of living or to toxic type of interventions that are encountered later in life. So, harmful basal ganglia neuronal changes that occur early in life could set the stage and shape the destiny of the individuals to the development of PD.

The dopamine neurons that are degenerated in PD have as their distinguishing feature long axons that project from the substantia nigra in the midbrain to the neostriatum in the forebrain region. One of the key sub-structures of the axon is cytoskeleton. Since they are involved in major cytoarchitectural changes during the development of the nigrostriatal dopamine neurons, the cytoskeleton and other associated molecules, including the kinases, are prime targets for modifications that will determine the outcome of the nigrostriatal dopaminergic neurons.

4.1. The involvement of cytoskeleton and alpha-synuclein as axonal constituents

The cytoskeleton proteins are important structures in the developmental and maintenance of the basal ganglia dopaminergic neurons. They support cellular shape, axonal and dendritic extensions, trafficking and transportation of macromolecules. More importantly, they allow the neurons to extend their reaches and influences far distances from the soma in the midbrain to the striatum in the forebrain region. So, the cytoskeleton serves to distinguish the new nigrostriatal dopaminergic neurons from the parent parochial cells and is the key components that enable the neurons to be functional; noting that the cell bodies may be correctly in place in the substantia nigra, but they will be non-functional without their far-reaching axons. So, by virtue of their relative cyto-architectural and functional significance, cytoskeleton synthesis and assembling ought to be one of the most vulnerable features affected by agents that interfere with the differentiation and proliferation of the far-reaching nigrostriatal dopaminergic neurons. Accordingly the molecules of the cytoskeleton protein classes, (i) microtubules, (ii) neurofilaments and (iii) microfilaments are seen as prime targets. Their vulnerability may help to explain why key markers of neurodegenerative disorders are mostly insoluble remnants of cytoskeleton protein. Lewy bodies, the major pathological marker for PD are composed principally of neurofilament proteins, alpha synuclein, actin-like protein, microtubules associated protein 2 (MAT 2), microtubules associated protein 5 (MAT 5), syaptophysin, tubulin (Giasson et al, 2000). Lewy bodies are also reactive for cytoskeletal protein kinases, calcium/calmodulin-dependent protein kinase (Iwatsubo et al, 1991), cyclin-dependent kinase 5 (Nakamura et al, 1997) and stress activated protein kinases (Giasson et al, 2000).

The microtubules include the subunits, (i) alpha-tubulin and beta-tubulin and (ii) polymerization regulator proteins that include microtubule associated protein 2 and 5 (MAP2 and MAP5). Microtubules span the length of axon and dendrites, serving as the track for macromolecular transport. They are the major component of mitotic spindle, an organelle that participates in cell division and are of importance in the differentiation of cells to form the nigrostriatal dopaminergic neuronal phenotype. Microtubules also play an important role in cell movement. The subunit, tubulin, synthesized in the cell body is actively transported down the axon, so they are relatively easy target for interfering molecules, such as colchicines. Moreover, the turnover of microtubules requires the polymerization and depolymerization of the molecule. This is a cyclic process that is more stable in mature dendrites and axons but is active in dividing cells, which again is a potential target for molecules, such as colchicines and vinblastine. So, the process that involves polymerization and depolymerization of microtubules is a weak link in the life of a far-reaching neuron during which modifications of a permanent nature can be made.

The neurofilaments are the most abundant fibrillar components of axon (Schwartz, 1991). They include the light (L), medium (M) and heavy (H) molecular weight neurofilament subunit proteins. Neurofilaments are oriented along the length of the axons, are most abundant in axons and are critical for axonal extension, a feature that enables the DA cell bodies in the substantia nigra to extend their axons to the striatum. So, neurofilament proteins form the 'backbones of the nigrostriatal DA neurons and interference with the protein will likely cause significant and permanent change.

Microfilaments are made up of globular subunits of (i) beta-actin and (ii) gamma-actin. Actin plays a major role in the function of growth cones and in dendritic spines. High concentrations occur in dendritic spines and they are located just underneath the plasmalemma, together with a large number of actin binding proteins, including spectrin-fodrin, ankyrin, talin and actinin. They play key role in motility of growth cone during development, the generation of specialized micro domains on the cell surface and in the formation of presynaptic and postsynaptic morphological specializations. They undergo cycles of polymerization and depolymerization (Kandel, Schwartz and Jessel, 2000).

Alpha-synuclein is also a likely prime target for prenatal toxins. It is a heat stable protein associated with synaptic vesicles and axonal terminals (Withers et al, 1997). It plays important roles in neurotransmission, synaptic organization and neuronal plasticity (George et al, 1995). Alpha-Synuclein is the major building block for the fibrillary component of Lewy's bodies (Pollannen et al, 1993), the major antigenic component of Lewy's bodies (Baba et al. 1997; Spillantini et al, 1997) and may be critical for the expression of PD symptoms (van Duinen et al, 1999). It is also a component of the thread-like structures seen in the perikarya of some neurons in the brainstem nuclei of the PD victims (Arima at al, 1998). It has been shown also that the association of alpha-synuclein with membrane promotes alpha synuclein aggregation (Lee et al. 2002) and that alpha-synuclein binds with dopamine transporters (Lee et al. 2001).

The interaction of the cytoskeleton proteins and other proteins of interest has been observed. For example, tubulin seeds the fibrillar form of alpha synuclein (Alim et al, 2002) and parkin has been shown to be a novel tubulin binding protein (Ren et al, 2003). It was also observed that 1-methyl-4-phenylpyridinium (MPP^+), the toxic metabolite of MPTP, reduced the synthesis of tubulin in PC12 cell model (Capelletti et al, 1999, Capelletti et al, 2000) and that MPP^+ inhibited tubulin polymerization (Capelletti et al, 2001), by specifically binding to tubulin in the microtubule lattice (Capelletti et al, 2005). Antibodies that recognize phosphorylated neurofilamant-M and neurofilaments-H also label Lewy's bodies, therefore the phosphorylation state of neurofilaments may be important in the formation of Lewy's bodies (Julien and Mushynski, 1998; Sternberger et al. 1983; Lee et al. 1987).

4.2. There may be a window of vulnerability for nigrostriatal dopamine neuronal sensitization

PD occurs in a relatively small number of the population, which may be so because a relatively short window of time exists during which the nigrostriatal DA neurons of the individual can be easily harmed. Such a window of vulnerability, we believe, is the period of differentiation, neurogenesis and migration of cells to form the nigrostriatal DA neurons, and this period occurs during gestational day 9-11 in mice. As mentioned above, the synthesis and laying down of cytoskeleton and neurotransmitter synthesis, storage, uptake and release capacities are likely the prime time during which the transforming cells are most vulnerable to toxic type of interference and inappropriate levels of metabolites and factors. So, idiopathic PD and some other degenerative disorders may have their origin in the fetus and the vulnerability may occur during pregnancy. This should not be seen as shifting the blame of having PD on pregnancy, but the fact is, pregnancy also produces the life and existence of the individual in the first place. So, the probability of having PD would be proportionate to the duration of the neurogenesis/neuronal development time, the number of pregnancy, the frequency by the individual encounter the toxic factor and the potency of the toxic encounter.

4.3. The susceptible stage may set the age of onset of PD and the severity of PD symptoms

If the rate of change is constant during the precipitating stage, it means that the more severe the sensitization, susceptible or vulnerable stage of affliction is, the earlier will the threshold reached for expressing the symptoms of PD. Thus, the age at which PD occurs may be directly related to the severity of the impairments that occur during the sensitization or the first stage affliction. So, juvenile PD may be marked by basal ganglia that were severely affected or were made less resilience by the changes that occur during the sensitization, susceptible or vulnerable stage of affliction. The individuas whose basal ganglia are less severely affected during the sensitization, susceptible or vulnerable stage may experience a delay in the expression of PD symptoms, since more harm will need to be made during the precipitating stage to reach the threshold at which PD symptoms will be seen. So individuals with the least affected nigrostriatal system during the susceptible stage are those that may live without the experiencing the symptoms of PD. In other words, the severity of the changes that occur during the sensitization, susceptible or vulnerable stage may very well predetermine the age at which PD symptoms will occur and the severity of the symptoms.

4.4. The number of NS DA neurons may also determine the susceptibility to PD

The proposed early exposures of the basal ganglia may reduce the number of NS neurons in a random pattern, among the population, so that the average individual possesses a normal population of, say 120,000 (120K) NS DA neurons and with various fractions of the population having values above and below the 120K. Thus, a bell-shaped frequency distribution pattern will exist, with some individuals represented at the far left of the curve, say with 30K or 25%. The individuals among the population who will most likely develop PD would be those endowed with a low (pre-threshold) population of 30K NS DA neuronal subset and PD will occur following a reduction of merely 6K neurons, to 20% of the mean. This low population number of neurons, similar to the marginally resilience neurons mentioned above, would constitute the 1st stage or the sensitization, susceptible or vulnerable stage, and contributes to the cause of PD. During the wear-and-tear of aging, that involves the reduction of NS DA neurons, individuals with the 30K number of NS DA neurons will be those most likely to develop PD symptoms and also at an early age (juvenile). This analogy could form the basis for the early-onset to late-onset PD cases. It may also explain the PD-like dispositions that are exhibited by the very old, due to the chronic reduction of NS DA neurons. The population at the right of the bell shape curve may be those that live to old ages without basal ganglia impairments.

4.5. The coincidental involvement of other neuronal sets with the NS neuronal changes

When the NS DA neurons are made susceptible during the early stage of life other neuronal groups may also be harmed by the modifying factor(s) and the coincidence will determine the occurrence of other symptoms with the symptoms of PD. The coincidental involvement may occur if the window of exposure or neurogenesis for the basal ganglia DA neurons overlap the period of neurogenesis for other neuronal sets, or the period of exposure to the interfering factor/factors is long enough to overlap the period of neurogenesis of all neuronal sets. If that is the case all the neuronal sets will be harmed by the interfering factor/factors. For example, if the nucleus basilis of Meynert acetylcholinergic neurons and the mesolimbic or mesocortical catecholaminergic neurons are affected, as proposed for the NS DA neurons, these other neuronal sets will be scared early in life and succumb to the wear-and-tear of aging later in life. Such co-incident may explain the comorbidity of

Alzheimer-like dementia as well as depression with the occurrence of PD. It is of interest, therefore, that the Guam amyotrophic lateral sclerosis-parkinsonism-dementia that may be caused by toxins from the cycad plant (Spencer, 1987), may involve the early damage to upper motor and lower neurons, NS DA neurons and nucleus basalis of Meynert neurons and that the failure of the neuronal sets later in life precipitates the triage of symptoms. This may involve a longer time for the early exposure, which is reasonable because the toxin in cycad was taken in as food. So, the impairments of various neuronal sets during the stage of neurogenesis and neuronal development may help to explain the variations and complexity of the PD related syndrome.

4.6. Agents that may cause neuronal susceptibility

Parkinson's disease was described by James Parkinson in 1817, almost two centuries ago. So, if external factors are involved in the cause of PD they were in the environment during those early times and the factors would be widely distributed since the occurrence of idiopathic PD is universal. Moreover, since aging is the key risk factor for having PD, PD can be seen as the outcome of the changes that occur during the wear-and-tear of aging. As mentioned above, the best scenario is that the changes in aging coupled with early events that render the nigrostriatal neurons susceptible. Several agents or conditions may be involved in causing the NS DA neurons to be susceptible because all that is required is for the factor to cause damage to dividing and developing neurons, and for the factors to be available during the critical stage of the birth of the NS DA neuronal phenotype. The deficiency and excesses of otherwise normal metabolites, such as momentary fetal hypoxia during the development of the NS DA neurons may be all that is required to trigger the sensitization, susceptible or vulnerable stage. There may also be excesses of normal metabolites, since high activity of cyclic AMP can block the induction of dopamine neurons (Hayes et al, 1995).

It is highly likely that the susceptible phase occurs over a short period, which may help to explain the relatively low incidence of PD. We have used the toxin, 1-methyl-4-phenyl-1,2,3,6-tetrahydropyridine (MPTP), to model the sensitization stage in the mice (Muthian et al, 2010), so structurally similar agents to MPTP that occur in nature could affect the basal ganglia long before the synthetic MPTP became available as a toxicant. It is proposed, also, that agents such as colchicine and vincristine that have been in use as medicine for over 2000 years could have played a role as a sensitization factor for PD. Colchicine is an alkaloid from the Lily family, including Autumn lily or Colchicum autumnale and of the saffron family, that is still used today, as food coloring and cosmetics. Vincristine is an alkaloid obtained from the periwinkle plant. These two compounds are not known to target the nigrostriatal dopamine neurons, however, they bind to tubulin and prevent the polymerization of tubulin to form microtubules. By doing so, they interfere with cell division and are known to arrest cell division in the metaphase stage. It means that these agents will interfere with the division of the newly proliferating nigrostriatal dopamine neurons if they are administered during the period of neurogenesis. They will also interfere with cellular transport, cell polarization, cell growth and axonal extension that depend on the integrity of cytoskeleton proteins. These features are especially important for a group of cells, such as the basal ganglia DA neurons that require their long axonal reaches to the striatum for their actions and effectiveness. By interfering with the assembling of the microtubules of the cells, colchicines and vincristine and now MPTP, via MPP^+, (Capelletti et al, 2005), will also impede and/or retard the new neurons from migrating to their place of destination in the substantia nigra, pars compacta. The phenomenon will also prevent the cells from extending their axons to their targets in the striatum. Since colchicines have been found to abolish retrograde transport in neurons resulting in the withdrawal of presynaptic terminals (Schwartz, 1991), these alkaloids will eventually result in cell death due to the lack of contact or contact inhibition. Today colchicines are used as a research tool and as a drug and the range of their toxicity is well known. Toxins, such as colchicines and vincristine are not disease specific, but they can cause a specific disease outcome based on the timing of their toxic effects to coincide with the vulnerable stage of a cellular substrate that underlie a specific disorder. For example, if a fetus is exposed to colchicines or vinblastine during the period of the neurogenesis and development of cells to produce the nigrostriatal dopaminergic phenotype, these neurons will be selectively harmed, and likely will result in PD later in life. If the effect of the toxin coincides with the birth of the nucleus basalis of Meynert neurons, Alzheimer's type dementia will occur. However, if the exposure time is extended to overlap both the birth of the nigrostriatal and acetylcholine neuronal sets the final symptoms will show parkinsonism and Alzheimer's like dementia.

4.7. Testing the prenatal sensitization, susceptibility or vulnerable concept

In studies designed to test the effects of toxin on the development of the midbrain neurons that are destined to become the nigrostriatal phenotype, we administered MPTP during the stage of neurogenesis, proliferation, migration and development of these DA cells. In the mouse, this period occurs during gestation day 9 - 11 and is marked by the appearance and maturation of TH-containing immunoreactive nigrostriatal neurons. The pregnant dams were treated with various dosages of MPTP or with phosphate buffered saline (PBS), as the control. We found that the dams treated with the 20 mg/kg and 30 mg/kg levels of MPTP, amounts that did not caused marked acute toxicity in the dams, caused very low to no full term pregnancy, suggesting that the higher dosage of MPTP may cause the pups to be aborted. For the 10 mg/kg of MPTP, however, the dams delivered normal looking pups, and this dosage was used to test the prenatal effects of MPTP.

4.7.1. Prenatal effects of MPTP on body weight, motor activity, TH and DA.

The outcome showed that the birth weights of pups born to dam that were exposed to prenatal 10 mg/kg of MPTP lagged behind the PBS control, but caught up within 4 weeks (Muthian et al, 2010). This recovery in birth weight and the appearance of the offspring indicated that they were in good physical health. The prenatal exposure to MPTP also reduced motor activity, measured as the total distance travelled, the movement time and the number of movements (Muthian et al, 2010) and Western blot detection showed that the exposure of the pregnant dams to MPTP at G9-11, that targeted the developing nigrostriatal dopamine neurons, reduced striatal tyrosine hydroxylase (TH) protein by 38%. DA and the metabolites of DA were also studied in the brain of the 12 week old C57BL/CJ mouse offspring following the prenatal exposure to10 mg/kg of MPTP or to PBS (Muthian et al, 2010). As shown in table 1, the prenatal exposure to MPTP reduced the concentrations of striatal dopamine (DA), homovanillic acid (HVA) and 3-methoxytyramine (3-MT) by 13.80%, 16.48% and 66.25%, respectively (Muthian et al, 2010). The level of dihydroxyphenylacetic acid (DOPAC) showed a slight increase (table 1).

	Dopamine and metabolites (ng/mg protein)			
Prenatal Treatments	DA [%]	DOPAC [%]	HVA [%]	3-MT [%]
PBS	157.3 ± 17.30 [0.0]	5.2 ± 0.76 [0.0]	18.2 ± 0.80 [0.0]	1.60 ± 0.20 [0.0]
MPTP	135.6 ± 4.80 [13.8]	5.9 ± .88 [+13.46]	15.2 ± 0.80 [16.48]	0.54 ± 0.12 [66.25]

Table 1. Effects of prenatal MPTP on striatial DA, DOPAC, HVA and 3-MT. C57BL/6J dams were treated with 10 mg/kg MPTP or with PBS during G8-G12 to target the developing nigrostriatal dopamine neurons in the fetus. The table shows the levels of DA, DOPAC, HVA and 3-MT in the striatum of the 12 weeks old offspring. MPTP reduced DA, HVA and 3-MT, as compared to the values for the PBS group.

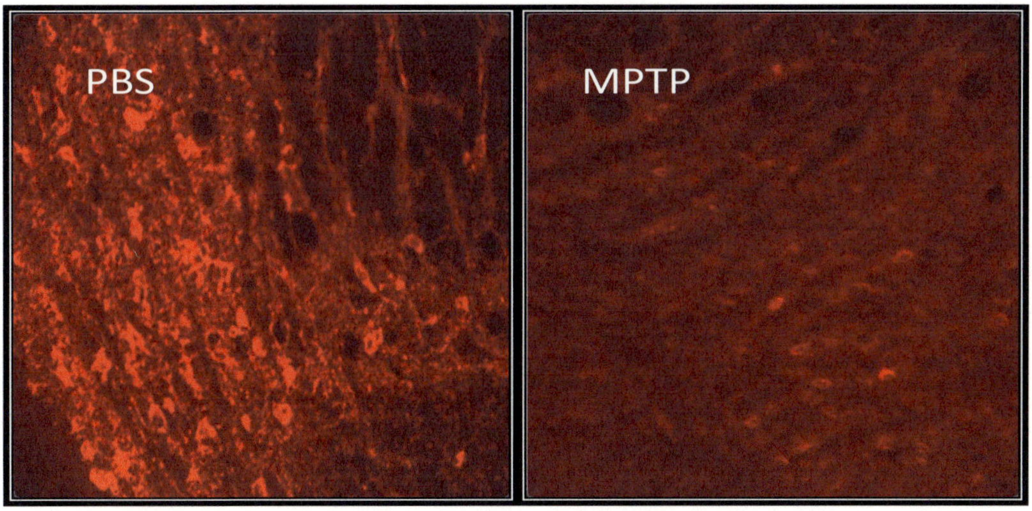

Figure 1. Substantia nigra, compacta of mice showing tyrosine hydroxylase immunoreactivity. The figure shows tyrosine hydroxylase (TH) immunoreactivity (I) in the substantia nigra compacta of a 12 weeks old mouse that was exposed to PBS (left) and one that was exposed to MPTP (right) in utero. The pregnant dam was treated during gestation days 8-12 and TH-I was determined in the 12 weeks old offspring.

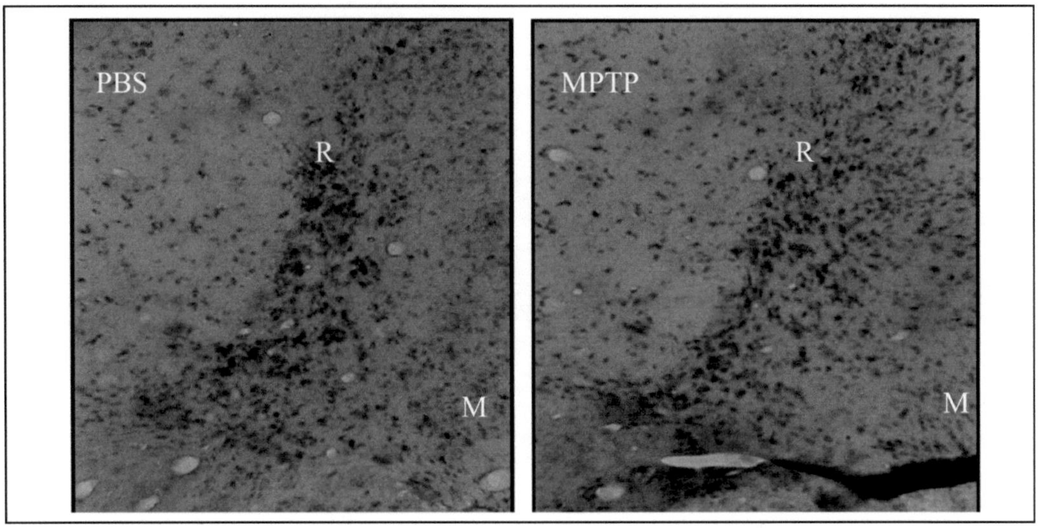

Figure 2. Nissl staining of the substantia nigra of mice exposed to prenatal PBS or MPTP. The Nissl staining highlights the cells (dots) of the substantia nigra, pars compacta. The overall morphology is closely similar, but the cellular composition of the PBS exposed mice are more concentrated within a defined zone in the compacta and with larger cells, as compared to the mice exposed to MPTP in which the smaller cells, especially within the rostro-medial (R-M) zone, are more abundant.

4.7.2. Prenatal MPTP on the in situ TH immunoreactivity in the substantia nigra

Figure 1 shows the effects of the prenatal exposure to MPTP on midbrain TH immunohistochemistry. Polyclonal antibodies against tyrosine hydroxylase (TH) were used to detect the changes that occurred in 12 weeks old mice offspring that were exposed to 10 mg/kg of MPTP, in utero, during G8-12 of the dam's pregnancy, when the midbrain neurons are developing the tyrosine hydroxylase phenotype. The results show that TH-like immunoreactivity was reduced in the midbrain substantia nigra of a mouse exposed to MPTP. The rostroventral section of the substantia nigra compacta was taken from horizontal slice of the mouse brain. The left section shows the TH immunoreactivity from a mouse offspring that was preexposed to PBS during G8-12 of the pregnant dam. The right section shows the TH inmmunoreactivity of a mouse offspring that was exposed to 10 mg/kg of MPTP during G8-12. The study shows that marked reduction of TH-I occurred in the mouse that was exposed in utero to MPTP (right).

4.7.3. Prenatal effect of MPTP on the Nissl Stained substantia nigra

The effect of prenatal exposure to MPTP on cellular distribution pattern in the substantia nigra, compacta of C57BL/CJ mice is shown in figure 2 as low magnification Nissl stained section of the 12 weeks old mice offspring. The differences in the cellular patterns for the PBS and the MPTP exposed animals were not marked, but cellular pattern seems to occur in the compacta zone for the PBS control as compared to the mouse that was exposed to MPTP, in which more scattered smaller cells can be seen in the medial (M) to rostral (R) zone of the substantia nigra (figure 1). The proportion of neurons to glia cells are unknown and are yet to be determined.

5. The inducing, precipitating or superimposing stage of the hypothesis

PD shares some characteristics with aging and the incidence of PD is higher in the aged individuals, but only a relatively small number of elders (about 0.3%) developed full-blown PD, therefore, since PD is sporadic it would appear that a predisposition exists for the disorder. The individuals that developed PD may have been predisposed or susceptible throughout their lives, and they develop PD symptoms when metabolic changes associated with getting older caused further harms to the nigrostriatal DA neurons and reduced the number of neurons. The precipitating effects may be due to various factors, such as changes that allow molecules that serve normal functions early in life to become toxic via direct or indirect ways, such as the production of toxic byproducts, for example. The exposure to

DA and Metabolites (ng/mg protein)	Prenatal Exposure.	Postnatal MPTP Challenges (mg/kg)			
		0 (PBS)	10	20	30 mg/kg
DA	PBS	157.3 ± 17.3 [0.0]	141.0 ± 5.50 [10.35]	34.5 ± 1.7 [78.06]	16.40 ± 2.0 [89.57]
	MPTP 10mg/kg	135.6 ± 4.80 [13.80]	48.0 ± 7.10 [69.96]	28.0 ± 2.0 [82.20]	3.95 ± 1.0 [97.49]
DOPAC	PBS	5.2 ± 0.76 [0.0]	6.00 ± 1.00 [15.38]	3.3 ± 0.4 [36.53]	1.95 ± 0.41 [62.5]
	MPTP 10mg/kg	5.9 ± 0.88 [+13.46]	1.04 ± 0.96 [80.0]	0.46 ± 0.58 [91.15]	0.41 ± 0.33 [92.11]
HVA	PBS	18.2 ± 0.80 [0.0]	17.5 ± 1.00 [3.85]	9.84 ± 0.6 [45.93]	6.0 ± 0.47 [67.03]
	MPTP 10mg/kg	15.2 ± 0.80 [16.48]	9.4 ± 0.66 [48.35]	8.3 ± 2.1 [54.39]	4.7 ± 0.70 [74.17]
3-MT	PBS	1.6 ± 0.20 [0.0]	1.2 ± 0.15 [25.0]	0.75 ± 12 [53.22]	0.54 ± 0.11 [66.25]
	MPTP 10mg/kg	0.54 ± 0.12 [66.25]	0.45 ± 0.11 [65.38)	0.32 ± 0.05 [80.0]	0.32 ± 0.06 [80.0]

Table 2. Postnatal effects of MPTP in mice offspring exposed to in utero MPTP or PBS. Effects of postnatal MPTP (10, 20, 30 mg/kg) on striatal DA, DOPAC, HVA and 3-MT in 12 weeks old mice offspring exposed to prenatal MPTP or PBS. The percent changes based on the normal PBS population levels are enclosed by brackets below the respective concentrations. The results show that postnatal MPTP was more effective in reducing DA and its metabolites in the offspring that were exposed to prenatal MPTP. However, for the 20 and 30 mg/kg doses of MPTP the significance of the postnatal, precipitating concept was masked because those doses of MPTP also markedly reduced DA and its metabolites in the prenatal PBS offspring.

exogenous toxic insults may also occur. This is represented by the outbreak of the 1919 encephalitis lethargic epidemic (Ravenholt et al, 1992) that precipitated PD symptoms among some of those that were affected by the encephalitis virus. Whether the inducing, precipitating or superimposing stage is due to metabolic changes or exposure to toxins, it should be noted that the effects do not have to be specific to cause the expression of the specific symptoms of PD, since the incidence during the first stage marks or sensitizes the nigrostriatal system, accordingly, any toxin or any change that can cause further harm to neurons, even in a general way, will affects those neurons that were made fragile.

5.1. Testing the inducing, precipitating or superimposing stage

We have shown that MPTP can be used to model the inducing, precipitating or superimposing stage. This was demonstrated in our studies in which we found that the postnatal administration of MPTP to 12 weeks old offspring, that were exposed *in utero* to MPTP earlier, during the developmental stage of the NS DA neurons, showed dramatically reduced levels of DA and its metabolites, as compared to similar mice that were exposed to the PBS treatment. The magnitude of the changes matches the level seen in PD, when compared with the normal population, or the PBS controls (table 2). The 10 mg/kg dosage of MPTP given to the mice that were exposed to prenatal MPTP caused the most dramatic reduction of DA and its metabolites, as compared to the PBS control (Table 2, column 3 vs. 4 showing values for prenatal PBS vs. prenatal MPTP). The 20 and 30 mg/kg of postnatal MPTP markedly reduced DA in the prenatal exposed MPTP mice, but these dose levels of MPTP also caused dramatic reductions of DA and its metabolites in the prenatal PBS mice, as well, so the differences between the prenatal MPTP and the prenatal PBS were not as dramatic (Fig 2, column 3 vs. 5 and 6 showing values for prenatal PBS vs. pre natal MPTP).

6. Analogy that depicts the two stages of affliction hypothesis

The two stages of affliction hypothesis for PD may be best illustrated by an analogy of a motor vehicle tire that was manufactured with a specific defect due to poor quality steel cords imbedded in the carcass or the body of the tire, during a critical period in the manufacture of the tire. The tire shows all of the characteristics of normal tires, but on exposure to the roadway the frictions that cause normal wear in tires turn out to cause serious failure in the defective tire. An inspection of the failed tire will show specific failure of the steel cords. The subtle imperfection that occurs during the manufacture of the tire may be seen as the sensitization factor that tags the tire for the specific type of failure that occurs under normal usage. In this scenario, such a normal tire usage may constitute the period for the precipitating stage, the tire serves to depict the human brain, the cords depict the nigrostriatal dopamine neurons with their far-reaching axonal projections, and the roadway-frictions represent the wear-and-tear of living that increases as a function of age. The two stages of afflictions or the sensitization-precipitating hypothesis for PD may also explain the discordance for PD in monozygotic twins. The life-long personality difference between monozygotic twins discordant for Parkinson's disease suggests that the process responsible for the disorders of PD has its inception early in life (Ward et al, 1983). The developmental personality of the member of the monozygotic twins who developed PD was found to be more introvert but since being an introvert is not usually abnormal within the population, it may be deduced that at least a second factor should be involved in causing the PD in the affected twin. The primary factor could be the early changes that render the nigrostrital DA neurons susceptible and also reflected or coincide with personality difference. The second factor for the disorder expression may be related to the regression in dopamine cells that occurs during aging (see McGree et al 1977).

7. Special cases of PD may involve early-life and multiple neuronal groups

The Guam amyotrophic lateral sclerosis-parkinsonism-dementia complex (ALS-PDC) may represent an incident of PD in which wide-scale neuronal damage occurred during the sensitization stage, and the wear-and-tear of living or the aberrations associated with aging take their toll later in life. In other words, the nigrostriatal dopaminergic neurons that were impaired during the fetal development degenerate to the threshold level that causes PD symptoms. Above threshold neuronal death also occurred for the nucleus basalis of Meynert acetylcholinergic neurons and cortical neurons involve in memory and cognition and caused the dementia phase of ALS-PDC syndrome (Oyanagi, 2005). The lower and upper motor neurons systems that control skeletal muscle contraction also died to cause the amyotrophic lateral sclerosis phase of the disorder. The theory is based on the report that the ALS-PDC or otherwise PDC-ALS is essentially the convergence of three disorders. Patients with PDC showed the signs of rigidity, tremor and bradykinesia (Oyanagi, 2005), the classical signs of Parkinson's disease as well as dementia (Oyanagi, 2005), the main sign of Alzheimer's disease. The ALS phase of the Guam ALS-PDC disorder has been reported to be essentially similar to those of classic ALS. Moreover 5% of the patients with ALS subsequently developed the total clinical symptoms of the ALS-PDC and 38% of the patients with PDC eventually developed the PDC-ALS syndrome (Elizan, et al, 1966; Oyanagi, 2005). So the PDC syndrome may be based on the exposure of the fetus to the cycad toxin during the period of the neurogenesis of both nigrostriatal DA neurons and nucleus basalis neurons. The duration of the toxic exposure of the patients may have been long enough to coincide with the neurogenesis and migration of the nigrostriatal DA neurons as well as the nucleus basalis of Meynert acetylcholinergic neurons. For the ALS patients, it is proposed that the exposure to the prenatal toxin coincides with the birth of upper and lower motor neurons and causing deleterious effects early in life that sensitized them to stress that occurred later in life. The higher 38 percent of patients with ALS may be matching to the longer neurogenesis and proliferation period for the related motor neurons and therefore longer fetal exposure time.

7.1. Proposed fetal basis for the Guam ALS-PDC disorder

The proposition that beta-methylaminoalanine (BMAA), a toxin found in flour produced from the Cycad plant and eaten as food, caused ALS-PDC (Spencer et al, 1987), is of interest.

It was also claimed that the basal ganglia symptoms were produced in monkeys fed BMAA (Spencer 1966), but this claim was disputed on the basis that the dosage used was far too high to represent the amounts that are eaten by human (Ince and Codd, 2005; McGree and Steele, 2011), and the disease produced in the monkeys was a classic acute toxicity model (Ince and Codd, 2005), rather than the progressing model of the ALS-PDC seen in the Guam patients. Moreover, the disease occurred in patients who had not used cycad products for many years (Sacks 1998), again suggesting the fetal basis for this ALS-PDC disorder. The risk of ALS-PDC was carried by migrants who had resided on Guam for the first 18 years of life (Ince and Codd, 2005), suggesting that early exposure is important for those who developed the ALS/PDC disorder, and the disorder takes over 35 years to develop, which is a very long time for a metabolic toxin to cause direct toxicity, and this also deviates from the short-term toxic models that have been presented.

It would be surprising that a major toxin consumed as a major source of food by several families would be so limiting in the number of individual within a family who were affected. In other words, if the ALS-PDC syndrome is due to a single-stage bout of toxic exposure, it would be expected that the toxin, which is ingested regularly as food, would affect a larger proportion of the group. So, it is apparently more reasonable to propose that the individuals that developed the ALS-PDC in Guam were exposed during the period of vulnerability of the nigrostriatal dopaminergic neurons, the nucleus basilis of Meynert acetylcholinergic neurons and the upper and lower motor neurons. They bourne the scar of the early exposure that pair with the changes that occur during aging to precipitate the ALS-PDC syndrome later in life. The sensitization-precipitation concept may be true also for the PD-like toxicity caused by MPTP in the later years of the 70s to the 80s. This may be so because not all individuals who were exposed to intravenous MPTP eventually developed full blown PD symptoms. Those that developed the symptoms of PD were probably predisposed with less resilient nigrostriatal neuronal set, and those that were spared had highly resilient nigrostriatal dopaminergic neurons. It means therefore, that most cases of PD may be caused by encounter made during the stage of neurogenesis and development of the nigrostriatal dopamine neurons, and that aging, the key risk factor for PD, precipitates idiopathic PD. The progressive nature of idiopathic PD may be based on the fact that aging is relenting and progressive in its own right.

8. S-adenosyl-L-methionine (SAM): A model precipitating factor for Parkinson's disease

S-adenosyl-L-methionine (SAM) is presented as a likely precipitating factor for PD. SAM is a naturally occurring and ubiquitous molecule derived from methionine and ATP (Cantoni 1953). It is one of the most reactive and important biochemical (Kotb and Geller, 1993), but its activity seems to be harnessed by the limits and the control placed on its synthesis. SAM is apparently synthesized on demand and rapidly utilized by several enzymes, as the biological methyl donor (Cantoni 1953), for trans-sulfuration reactions and in the synthesis of polyamine (Andres and Cederbaum 2005). As the biological methyl donor, SAM is the co-factor for several methyl transferases, including catechol-O-methyl transferase (COMT) and indole amine methyl transferase. COMT transfers the methyl of SAM to dopamine (DA) to produce 3-methoxytyramine and to norepinephrine (NE) to produce normetaphrene and by doing so SAM terminates the synaptic activities of DA and NE, via irreversible reactions. SAM also serves to methylate N-acetyl-serotonin, via indoleamine methyltransferase to form melatonin and in the process may deplete serotonin (5-HT). These are major metabolic processes since DA, NE and 5-HT are important in synaptic transmission and in behavior (Agnoli et al, 1976) and are reported to be depleted in PD. So, SAM is a highly reactive endogenous molecule.

The injection of SAM into the cerebral ventricle of rodents produced symptoms that are similar or identical to those described for PD, including hypokinesia, rigidity, tremors (Charlton and Way 1978), the loss of DA, loss of striatal and substantia nigra tyrosine hydroxylase (Charlton, 1990; Charlton and Crowell, 1995; Crowell et al, 1993) and loss of neurons in the substantia nigra (Charlton and Mack, 1994).The PD-like changes that occurred following the cerebral ventricular administration of SAM are based on very logical and mechanistic grounds, since SAM reacts avidly with L-dopa and DA and reduced DA. More importantly, the loss of DA is the hallmark of PD disease, and the methylation of DA at the synapse (Axelrod, 1965) terminates the neurotransmitter activity of DA; a process that irreversibly destroys the dopamine molecule by covalently converting it to 3-methoxytyramine. SAM also drives the synthesis of phosphotidylcholine (PTC) (Hirata et al, 1981) that is accompanied with increases in lyso-PTC (Lee and Charlton 2001), a potent membrane damaging surfactant. It has been shown also, that SAM interacted with and methylated DA receptor protein and inhibited DA receptor binding (Lee and Charlton, 2004). In addition, the carboxylmethylation of protein, including DA receptor protein, by SAM, generates methanol (Axelrod and Daly, 1965), formaldehyde and formic acid (Lee et al 2008), reactive byproducts that can cause irreversible and accumulative damaging changes to cells and cellular constituents. Although the biological role of methanol, formaldehyde and formic acid are not viewed with much significance, these molecules are likely to be of primordial origin, helping to shape the destiny of life. They are produced in the body and are extremely reactive. The activity of SAM is also increased during aging (Mays and Borek 1973; Stramentinoli et al, 1977; Gharib et al, 1982; Sellinger et al, 1988), a critical period for cellular attrition and a stage of life during which the symptoms of idiopathic PD are seen. Today SAM is well studied as the major driver of the epigenetic modification of various genes. The biochemical control that SAM exhibited is remarkable on the basis that SAM is the limiting factor for dozens of methyltransferases, so any increase or decrease in the level of SAM serves as a key driving force for most methylation reactions.

8.1. Common markers exist for methylation and parkinsonism

A review of the results from various laboratories, include our own, shows that various biochemical, functional, anatomical and other markers are common to PD and to the methylation process (Table 3). Metabolites and byproducts of SAM, such as N-methyl dopamine, 3,4-dimethoxy-dopamine, N-methylsalsolinol (Maruyama, et al, 1996; Naoi et al, 2002; Matsubara et al, 2002) and harman and norharman (Kuhn, et al, 1996) are elevated in

Biological Events	PD relevance	Effect on/of SAM
Biochemical changes		
Decreased dopamine	Yes	Yes
Decreased norepinephrine	Yes	Yes
Decreased serotonin	Yes	Yes
Decreased melanin	Yes	Yes
Decreased tyrosine hydroxylase	Yes	Yes
Increased Ach activity	Yes	Yes
Increased HVA/DA	Yes	Yes
Increased DIMPEA	Yes	Yes
Functional defects		
Hypokinesia	Yes	Yes
Tremors	Yes	Yes
Rigidity	Yes	Yes
Abnormal posture	Yes	Yes
Anatomical impairments		
Nigrostriatal damage	Yes	Yes
Loss of DA/TH neurons	Yes	Yes
Other markers		
Older ages	More prevalent	High activity of SAM
L-dopa	Alleviates	Depletes SAM
Methionine	Aggravates	Increased SAM
N-methyl tetrahydroisoquinoline	Causes/in PD brain	SAM metabolite
Methyl beta carboline	Causes	SAM metabolite
MPTP/MPP+	Causes	Enhances methylation
N-methyldopamine	Found in	SAM metabolite
N-methylsalsolinol	Found in	SAM metabolite
Homocysteine	Found in	SAM metabolite
MPP^+	Aggravates	Increased SAM activity
Manganese	Aggravates	Increased SAM activity
Lyso-phosphotidylcholine	PD-like effects	Increased by SAM
Nicotinamide-N-methyl-transferase	High in CSF	SAM is the cofactor

Table 3. Many biological changes seen in PD correspond with the effects of SAM. The table shows the parallel relationship between changes associated with Parkinson's disease and with the effects and biochemical activities of S-adenosyl-L-methionine and its metabolites. A one-one relationship is shown in the activities listed.

the CSF of PD patients and homocysteine (Lee et al, 2005) may cause PD like toxic changes. In addition, methyl-beta-carboline was reported to cause PD-like changes (Collins, et al. 1992; Gearhart et al, 1997). Furthermore, it has been shown that the tissues of PD patients methylate nicotinamide greatly higher than tissues of the control patients (Willams et al, 1993); and that nicotinamide methylation is proposed to be a key factor in the development of degenerative diseases (Williams and Ramsden, 2005). The enzyme, nicotinamide-N-methyltransferase, that transfers the methyl group from SAM to nicotinamide, was shown to be high in the CSF of PD patients (Aoyama et al, 2001) and N-methyl-nicotinamide was also higher in the brain of PD victims as compared to the control (Williams and Ramsden, 2005). So, as shown, many biological changes seen in PD correspond with the effects of SAM, its enzymes and its metabolites (table 3).

8.2. Actions and effects that support the role of SAM as a precipitation factor in PD

If a secondary precipitating factor is associated with PD, it would more likely fits as a toxic metabolite that is associated with aging. Such a metabolite would be expected to be very reactive. It would show age-related increases in activity, would have a narrow index of safety so that even slight increases would cause toxic reactions. It should react with normal biochemicals that are critically needed on a moment-by-moment basis for the maintenance of essential functions. Moreover, the metabolite should react with biochemical that are found to be modified during the course of PD, for example, DA that is depleted in PD and which is an avid methyl acceptor. In addition, the mode of reactivity of the metabolite should explain others changes that are related to the degenerative disease process, such as the effective therapy for PD and the development of tolerance to the therapeutic agent. So, an evaluation of S-adenosyl-L-methionine (SAM), the biological methyl donor, based on the above criteria, indicates that it fits the role of a precipitating factor for PD. Again, it is an endogenous molecule, its activity is increased during aging, it is very reactive, it has a narrow index of safety, it controls the metabolism of specific chemicals that are modified in PD, the major drug for PD, which is L-dopa, reacts avidly with SAM and L-dopa, in turn, induced methionine adenosyl transferase, the enzyme that produces SAM (Benson et al, 1993; Zhoa et al, 2001). Moreover, as mentioned above, several SAM-induced changes seem to be associated with the neuronal degeneration and many of the biochemical changes that occur in PD.

8.2.1. Age-dependent increases in SAM-dependent methylation

The activities of SAM, denoted by increases in its synthesis and utilization, are increased during aging. This has been reported as, an age-related increase in methionine-adenosyl transferase, the enzyme that produces SAM, increases of various methyl transferases, and the accumulation in products of SAM-dependent methylation reactions, including homocysteine and adenosine (Mays et al 1973; Stramentinoli et al, 1977; Sellinger et al 1988; Gharib et al 1982). It should be noted that a decrease in the absolute concentration of SAM in rats was reported to be related to aging (Baldessarini and Kopin, 1966) but the reduction was apparently due to increases in the turnover of SAM that also occurred during aging (Stramentinoli et al, 1977).

8.2.2. SAM depletion of biogenicamines may occur in PD

In the presence of catechol-O-methyltransferase and other transferases SAM serves as a cofactor in the methylated metabolism of several biogenic amines, including DA and norepinephrine, by donating its reactive methyl group mainly to receptive hydroxyl of the molecular ring and the nitrogen of the ethylamine side chain (Axelrod, 1965). SAM dependent methylation is the most important mechanism in mammals for the inactivation of catecholamine (Lambrosse et al 1958, Axelrod et al, 1965), consequently SAM is an important factor in controlling the neuronal levels of the biogenic amines. The decreased levels of DA (Hornykiewicz, 1966), norepinephrine (Erhinger and Hornykiewicz, 1960) and serotonin (Bernheimer et al, 1961) observed in PD could be explained by an increase in the methylation of DA, norepinephrine and of N-acetyl-serotonin. The methylation of DA may also explain the increase ratio of homovanillic acid (HVA) to DA (HVA/DA) in PD and the increased level of 3,4-dimethoxyphenylethylamine, the dimethoxy metabolite of DA, that was reported to be contained in the urine of PD patients. More importantly, the DA derived alkaloid, N-methyl-(R)-salsolinol, was shown to occur in the human brain, accumulates in the nigrostriatal system and may play a role in PD (Naoi et al, 2002). An increase SAM-dependent methylation may also help to explain the pharmacology of L-dopa, in treating the symptoms of PD, because L-dopa is not only converted to DA, but it also reacts avidly with SAM, and depletes SAM. SAM dependent regulation of biogenicamines is achieved by methylated catabolism as well as by increasing synthesis, because it has been shown that preincubation with SAM caused activation of tyrosine hydroxylase in the corpus striatum of rats (Mann and Hill, 1983). These and other outcomes suggest that SAM is functioning both intra- and extra-neuronal, therefore its bio-availability at specific sites should be critical in determining the up or down regulation of the activity of biogenicamines. SAM activation of tyrosine hydroxylase (Mann and Hill, 1983) may help to explain the increase in DA turnover that occurs in PD. An increase in the methylation of L-dopa and DA will shunt tyrosine toward the production of L-dopa and L-dopa toward the production of DA, thus, tyrosine will be shunted away from the synthesis of melanin, a process that may help to explain the reduction of melanin in the substantia nigra of PD patients: noting that melanin is a product of tyrosine. Likewise, SAM also methylates phosphotidylethanolamine to produce phosphotidylcholine and phosphotidylcholine, in turn, is metabolized to generates choline molecules for the synthesis of acetylcholine. So, an increase in methylation could conceivable increase the level of acetylcholine and acetylcholinergic activity that occurred in PD, and which may form the basis for the utility of anticholinergic agents in the treatment of PD symptoms.

8.2.3. Mechanisms and selectivity of SAM for the basal ganglia

Conditions that increase the rate of methylation, for example aging (Sellinger et al 1988), may precipitate PD in individuals with susceptible DA neuronal population. In individuals with the normal complement of substantia nigral DA neurons the same level of methylation may represent an age-dependent normal regression of cell population, because the critical cell level that will result in PD would not be reached. Thus, the final effects of an increase in methylation in persons with normal populations of DA neurons would be different degrees of aging. Besides aging, other factors that facilitate an increase in methylation ought to be emplaced. It turns out that (i) the chemistry of the basal ganglia, (ii) the anatomical and physical state of the basal ganglia and (iii) the functions that are controlled by the basal ganglia coexist in a cooperative way to facilitate the uniqueness of SAM as the methyl donor and as a putative precipitating factor for PD.

For the chemistry of the basal ganglia, the methylation of DA and the methylation of phosphotidylethanolamine may be of major importance. First, the methylation of DA by SAM depletes DA at the synaptic cleft. This is an irreversible reaction that also generates 3-methoxytyramine, a metabolite that has been shown to competes with DA for its receptor binding (Charlton and Crowell, 2000). So, the reaction of SAM with DA and the generation of an competing metabolite will not only depletes DA, but also will interfere with the binding of DA to its receptors, which is consistent with a SAM-induced dopaminolytic state. SAM also methylates phosphotidylethanolamine to produce phosphotidylcholine, and, as mentioned above, to produce choline for the synthesis of acetylcholine. In addition, phosphotidylcholine is readily hydrolyzed to form the toxic surfactant, lyso-phosphotidylcholine (Lee et al, 2001; 2005). The reaction is also relevant on the basis that lyso-phosphotidylcholine is a potent surface-active agent that will damage cellular vesicles and nerve ending, and can contribute to the progression of the degeneration that occurs in PD. The biochemical peculiarity of the basal ganglia, therefore, includes the fact that the neostriatum contains large quantities of L-dopa, DA and norepinephine that are avid methyl acceptors, so they utilize high levels of SAM. SAM is also required for the methylation of phospholipid and the synthesis of acetylcholine, so the neostriatum is a high utility site of SAM, or a chemical 'sink' for, SAM.

The precise functions of the basal ganglia marked it for visible impairments. The basal ganglia dopaminergic system controls precise articulation of the hands, finger, lips and whole body to support emotional expression, gesture and feelings. Therefore in the awaking human the neostriatum is constantly under stress to maintain the delicately balanced and fine-tuned processes that it controls, so slight impairments of the nigrostriatal system will upset the postural balances and precise muscle regulations and will cause visible impairments, that are seen as PD, even when such a degree of impairment or degeneration would not be physically obvious if occurred in other systems. SAM-related age-related changes may also affect vision and hearing, but the changes in the quality of life are not of the same magnitude as seen when the basal ganglia is impacted.

The anatomical or physically states of the basal ganglia also make this structure very accommodative to the effects of an increase in SAM, because SAM, which is very water soluble, will accumulate in the cerebral spinal fluid (CSF). In the CSF SAM is in close proximity to the neostriatum, which courses along and protruded into the lateral ventricle and contains the sensitive dopamine nerve terminals. Studies have shown that the administration of SAM into the lateral ventricle damaged the delicate ependymal cell barrier that separates the CSF from the caudate nucleus neuronal environment. By doing so, SAM gained access to the neostriatum, where it can deplete DA (Crowell et al, 1993), can methylate phospholipids (Lee and Charlton 2001) and DA receptor protein (Lee et al, 2004) and generate methanol, formaldehyde and formic acid (Lee et al, 2008) that are damaging to nigrostriatal dopamine nerve endings. These metabolites, especially formaldehyde will result in permanent changes to the dopaminergic neurons. Interestingly, in a more recent study, we found that the co-administration of a retrograde neuronal tracer with SAM into the lateral ventricle caused the labeling of cells in the substantia nigra, indicating that molecules placed in the lateral ventricle can gain access to the caudate nucleus DA nerve endings.

The increase in methylation can caused other significant changes, for example, the utilization of SAM imposes a great demand on ATP, because for every mole of DA methylated at the 3-OH and 4-OH positions 2 moles of ATP are utilized to replenish the utilized SAM and for every mole of phosphotidylethanolamine that is methylated to form phosphotidylcholine 3 mole of ATP are required to replenish SAM. Furthermore, the carboxyl methylation of protein by SAM will increase the isoprenylation of the proteins and each farnesyl molecule that is utilized requires 3 moles of ATP for its synthesis and each geranyl-geranyl requires 4 moles of ATP for its synthesis. So, an increased methylation will require increased production of ATP, which increases oxygen utilization and the probability of generating reactive oxygen species. In addition, 1 mole of potentially toxic homocysteine and 1 mole of adenosine may be produced for every mole of SAM utilized, and huge amounts of adenosine will be produced as a result of the metabolism of ATP to replenish SAM. The depletion of ATP may be relevant in this connection, because inhibition of mitochondrial oxidation and ATP reduction are proposed to be involved in the actions of MPTP or MPP^+. It is well understood that SAM-dependent methylation is a normal physiological process, so for one to imagine how SAM may be involved in PD it should be understood that the symptoms of PD are due directly to dopamine biochemical deficiency and indirectly to the neuronal degeneration. This is so because drugs, such as L-dopa and DA receptor agonists relieve the tremors and other symptoms of PD, in spite of the fact that the permanent neuronal degeneration remains. Furthermore, the syndrome of PD wax-and-wane, which, cannot be explained by the existence of a permanent degenerated neuronal set. These examples show that the symptoms of PD, such as tremor and freezing, are striatal biochemical deficiency symptoms, due to the loss of dopamine as a result of the neuronal degeneration.

In spite of the doubts about the methylation concept, it is of interest that most of the other hypotheses concerning the genesis of PD cannot explain many of the changes that are seen in PD. One-methyl-4-phenyl-1,2,3,6-tetrahydropyridine (MPTP) and 6-hydroxyl-dopamine (6-OHDA) serve as the most important chemical models for PD. Their efficacies are mostly related to the targeted nigrostriatal cell death, but these agents do not cause changes that reflect the whole spectrum of PD symptoms. For example, MPTP does not cause PD-like symptoms in the rat, which also has a nigrostriatal dopamine system, but SAM does (Crowell et al, 1992; Charlton and Mack, 1994).

9. Conclusion

The abberrations that cause the nigrostriatal degeneration that result in Parkinson's disease are unknown. Since about 90-95% of all cases of PD are not due to genetic changes, it means that the environment plays a major role in the cause of PD. The environment is not restricted to the toxins that might be involved, but includes the biochemical melieu that the nigrostriatal cells encounter from their origin to the outcome that causes them for die. So, the encounter with inappropriate biochemicals and inappropriate levels of the appropriate biochemicals may occur, and the outcome will vary and will be restricted to the nigrostriatal neurons or will involve other neuronal sets. This type of encounter will produce the syndrome that are eventually expressed and may include symptoms related to nigrostriatal damage only, but may be accompanied with other syndrome. So the expression of symptoms in addition to the classical PD other symptoms, suggests that nigrostriatal neuronal impairment may be accompanied with the impairments of other neuronal groups. These may include the basal nucleus of Meynert acetylcholinergic neurons that are degenerated in Alzheimer's disease (AD) and the upper and lower motor neurons that are involved in the cause of amyotrophic lateral sclerosis (ALS). So, the existence of the Guam amyotrophic lateral sclerosis-parkinsonism dementia complex (ALS-PDC, suggests that the factors that cause PD are not specific for the nigrostriatal neurons, but will affect other neuronal groups, as well.

For PD, it is suggested that the nigrostriatal dopaminergic neurons were exposed by chance encounter during a vulnerable stage of development of the neuronal set. Since aging is the key risk factor for PD, it also means that at least two stages of afflictions are involved in the cause of PD. Evidence and circumstance suggest that the first stage occurs in utero during the neurogenesis and development of cells to form the substantia nigra dopaminergic phenotype. The neuronal set is harmed in a subtle way that does not cause visual symptoms, but the sub-threshold effects weakened the resilience of the neurons so that the stress encounter during the course of living causes further harm to the already affected neurons and precipitates the symptoms of PD. So, the first impairment may occur during the neurogenesis and development of the nigrostriatal dopamine neurons by inappropriate levels of regulatory molecules or by toxins. An increased activity of cyclic-AMP-dependent protein kinase A, for example, may antagonize the signal for sonic hedgehog protein and blocked the induction of dopamine neurons (Hayes et al, 1995). The exposure to alkaloids, such as colchicine or vinblastine may also occur, and these alkaloids may interfere with the development of the cytoskeleton, with long-term and sub-threshold levels of effects. The stress of aging that causes globally deteriorating change will then take a toll on these low resilient neuronal sets to precipitate the symptoms of PD. The prenatal and postnatal effects can also explain the occurrence of juvenile PD, which would involve the substantia nigral dopamine neurons that were affected in ways that make them less resilient and more sensitive to age-related stress, so a short course of living would be enough to precipitate the symptoms of PD in the young individual. The Guam ALS-PDC cases are proposed to be caused by the exposure to the Cycad toxin during the neurogenesis and development of the nigrostriatal dopamine neurons, the basal neucleus of Meynert acetylcholinergic neurons and upper and lower motor neurons. The exposure caused subthreshold harms to those neuronal sets and they failed before other major groups of neurons during the course of aging.

The hypothesis that neurodegenerative disorders, such as PD and others have their origin in the womb is in line with normal physiology, since the lives of all mammals have their origin in the womb. If the hypothesis is tested to be true further investigation will identify the specific agents and/or the mechanisms that may be involved in the sensitization stage and measures could be adapted to protect the vulnerable neuronal groups during critical stages of fetal development.

Author details

Clivel G. Charlton
Meharry Medical College, USA

Acknowledgement

The author wishes to thank Gladson Muthian, Ph.D., Lemuel Dent, MD., MS; Veronica Mackay, B.S., Marquitta Smith, B.S. and Brenya Griffin, B.S. for their support of science in our laboratory. Supported by NIH NINDS R21NS049623, RO1NS28432 and R01NS31177 and Bernard Crowell, Jr. MD, Ph.D., Little Rock AR.

10. References

[1] Agnoli, A., Andreoli, V., Casacchia, M., and Cerbo, R. Effect of S-adenosyl-L-methionione (SAM-e) upon depressive symptoms. J. Psychiar. Res. 13: 43-54, 1976.

[2] Alim, MA., Hossain. MS., Arima, K., Takeda, K., Izumiyama, Y., Nakamura, M., Kaji, H., Shinoda, T., Hisanaga, S., Ueda, K., Tubulin seeds alpha-synuclein fibril formation. J. Biol. Chem. 277(3): 2112-2117, 2002.

[3] Alvord Jr., EC., Forno, LS., Kusske, JA., Jaufman, RJ., Rhodes, JS., Goetowski, CR. The pathology of parkinsonism: Comparison of degeneration in cerebral cortex and brainstem. Adv. Neurol. 5:175-193, 1974.

[4] Andres, A and Cederbaum, AI. Antioxidant properties of S-adenosyl-L-methionine in Fe2+-initiated oxidants. Free Radical Biology & Med. 36 (10): 1303-1316, 2004.

[5] Aoyama, K., Matsubara, K., Konda, M., Murakawa, Y., Suno, M., Yamashita, S., Yamaguchi, S., and Kobayashi, S. Nicotinamide-N-methyl transferase is higher in the lumbar cerebrospinal fluid of patients with Parkinson's disease. Neurosci. Lett. 298: 78-80, 2001.

[6] Arima, K., Ueda, K., Sunohara, N. et al. Immunoelectron-microscope demonstration of NACP/alpha-synuclein-epitopes on the filamentous component of Lewy bodies in Parkinson's disease and in dementia with Lewy's bodies. Brain Res. 808: 93-100, 1998.

[7] Axelrod, J. and Daly, J. Pituitary gland: Enzyme formation of methanol from S-adenosyl- methionine. Science 150: 892-893, 1965.

[8] Axelrod, J. The metabolism, storage and release of catecholamine. Recent Prog. In Hormone Res. 21: 597-619, 1965.

[9] Baba, M., Nakajo, S., Tu, P. et al. Aggregation of alpha–synuclein in Lewy's bodies of sporadic Parkinson's disease and dementia with Lewy's bodies. Am. J. Pathol. 152: 879-884, 1997.

[10] Baldessarini, RJ. and Kopin, IJ. S-adenosylmethionine in brain and other tissues. J. Neurochem. 13: 769-777, 1966.
[11] Benson, R., Crowell, B., Hill, B., Doonquah, K. and Charlton, C. The effects of L-dopa on he activity of methionine adenosyltransferase: Relevance to L-dopa therapy and olerance. Neurochem. Res. 18 (3): 325-330, 1993.
[12] Bernheimer, H., Birkmayer, W. and Hornykiewicz, O. Verteilung des 5-hydroxytamin serotonin) im gehirn des menschen und sein verhaltan bei patienten mit Parkinson syndrom. Klin. Ther. Wschr. 39:1056-1059. 1961.
[13] Bon, MA., Jansen, EN., DeVos, RA. and Vermes, I. Correlates of Parkinson disease: Apolipoprotein-E and cytochrome P450 2D6 genetic polymorphism. Neurosci. Lett. 266(2):149-151, 1999.
[14] Cantoni, GL. S-adenosylmethionine: a new intermediate formed enzymatically from L-methionine and adenosine-triphosphate. J. Biol. Chem. 204: 403-416, 1953.
[15] Capelletti, G., Maggioni, MG. and Maci, R. Influence of MPP+ on the state of tubulin polymerization in NGF-differentiated PC12 cells. J. Neurosci. Res. 56: 28-35, 1999.
[16] Capelletti, G., Maggioni, MG. and Maci, R. Role of microtubules in the genesis of MPTP neurotoxicity. In: *Neurotoxic Factors in Parkinson's Disease and Related Disorders*. Eds: Storch, A. and Collins, MA., pp 45-48, Kluwer Academic/Plenum Publishers, New York.
[17] Capelletti, G., Pedrotti, B., Maggioni, MG. and Maci, R. Tubilin polymerization is directly affected by MPP+ in vitro. Cell Biol. Int. 25: 981-984, 2001.
[18] Capelletti, G., Surrey, T. and Maci, R. The parkinsonism producing MPP+ affects microtubule dynamics by acting as a destabilizing factor. FEBS Letters 579: 4781-4786, 2005.
[19] Casanova, M., Deyo, DF. and Heck, HA. Covalent binding of inhaled formaldehyde to DNA in the nasal mucosa of Fisher 344 rats: analysis of formaldehyde and DNA by high performance liquid chromatography and provisional pharmacokinetic nterpretation. Fund. Appl. Toxicol. 12: 397-417, 1989.
[20] Charlton, C. and Crowell, B. Striatal dopamine depletion, tremors, and hypokinesia ollowing the intracranial injection of S-adenosylmethionine. Mol. and Chem. Neuropath. 26: 269-281, 1995.
[21] Charlton, CG., Mack, J. Substantia nigra degeneration and tyrosine hydroxylase depletion caused by excess S-adenosylmethionine in the rat brain: Support for an excess methylation hypothesis for parkinsonism. Mol. Neurobio. 9: 149-61, 1994.
[22] Charlton, CG. and Crowell, B. The effects of metabolites of DA on locomotor activities and dopamine receptor binding in rats: Relevance to the side effects of L-dopa. Life Sci. 66 (22): 2159-2171, 2000. Hormone Res. 21: 597-619, 1965.
[23] Charlton, CG. (1990). A parallel relationship between Parkinson's Disease and excess of S-adenosylmethionine-dependent biological methylation in the brain. *Basic, Clinical and Therapeutic Aspects of Alzheimer's and Parkinson's Disease.* Vol. 1. Cpt. 65. Plenum Press. N.Y.
[24] Charlton, CG. and Way, EL. Tremor induced by S-adenosy1-L- methionine: possible relation to L-dopa effects. J. Pharm. Pharmacol. 30: 819-820, 1978.

[25] Charlton, CG and Crowell, B. Striatal dopamine depletion, tremors and hypokinesia following the intracranial injection of S-adenosylmethionine: A possible role for hypermethylation on Parkinsonism. Mol. and Chem. Neuropath. 26:269-284, 1995.

[26] Charlton, CG. 1-Methyl-4-phenylpyridinium (MPP+) but not 1-methyl-4-phenyl-1,2,3,6-tetrahydropyridine (MPTP) serves as methyl donor for dopamine: A possible mechanism of action. J. Geriat. Psychia. Neurol. 5(2): 114-118, 1992.

[27] Christensen, D., Idanpann-Heikkila JJ., Guilgaud, G. and Kayser, V. The antinociceptive effects of combined systemic administration of morphine and the glycine/NMDA receptor antagonist, (+)-HA966, in a rat model of peripheral neuropathy. Br. J. Pharmacol. 125(8): 1641-1650, 1998.

[28] Chu, N., Hochberg, F., Calne, D. and Olanow, C. Neurotoxicology of manganese. In: *Handbook of Neurotoxicolog*, Eds: Chang L. and Dyer, R. Mercel Dekker, New York, pp91-103, 1995.

[29] Crowell, B., Benson, R., Shockley, D. and Charlton, CG. S-adenosyl-methionine decreases motor activity in the rat: Similarity to Parkinson's disease-like symptoms. Behav. and Neural Biology 59: 186-193, 1993.

[30] Dauer, W., Kholodilov, N., Vila, M., Trillat, AC., Goodchild, R., Larsen, KE., Staal, R., Tieu, K., Schmitz, Y., Yuan, CA., Rocha, M., Jackson-Lewis, V., Hersch, S., Sulzer, D., Przedborski, S., Burke, R. and Hen, R. Resistance of alpha-synuclein null mice to the parkinsonian neurotoxin MPTP. Proc. Natl. Acad. Sci., USA, 99:14524-14529, 2002.

[31] Davis, GC., Williams, AC., Markey, SP., Elbert, MH., Caine, ED., Reichert, CM. and Kopin, IJ. Chronic Parkinsonism secondary to intravenous injection of meperidine analogues. Psychiatry Res. 1: 249-254, 1979.

[32] Eadie, MJ. The pathology of certain medullary muclei in parkinsonism. Brain. Res. 86: 781-790, 1963.

[33] Egensperger, R., Kosel, S., Schnopp, NM. et al. Association of the mitochondria tRNA (A4336G) mutations with Alzheimer and Parkinson's disease. Neuropathol. Appl. Neurobiol. 23: 315-321, 1997.

[34] Ehringer, H. and Hornykeiwicz, O. Verteilung von noradrenalin unddopamin (3-hydroxytyramin) im gehirn des menscen und ihr verhalten bei erkrankungen des extra-phyramidalen systems. Klin-ther. Wschr. 38: 1236-1239. (cited in Scultz, 1960).

[35] Elble, RJ., Hughes, L. and Higins, C. The syndrome of senile gait. J. Neurol. 239: 71-75, 1992.

[36] Elble, RJ., Hughes, L., Higins, C. and Colliver, J. Stride-dependent changes in the gait of older people. J. Neurol. 238: 1-5, 1991.

[37] Elble, RJ. The role of aging in the clinical expression of essential tremors. Exp. Gerontol. 30: 337-347, 1995.

[38] Elizan, TS., Hirano, A., Abrams, BM., Need, RL., vanNuis C. and Kurland, LT. Amylotrophic lateral sclerosis and parkinsonism-dementia complex of Guam. Arch. Neurol. 14: 256-368, 1966.

[39] Foix, C. and Nicolesco, J. Overview of morphological changes in Parkinson's disease. Mason, Paris 1925. (Cited in Hillinger K. Adv. Neurology 45:1-18. 1986.)

[40] Forno, LS. And Norvill, RL. Ultrastructure of Lewy bodies in the stellate ganglion. Acta Neuropathol. 34: 183-197, 1976.
[41] Gasser, T., Wszolek, ZK., Oehlmann, R. et al. A susceptibility locus for Parkinson's disease on chromosome 2p13. Nat. Genet. 18: 262-265, 1998.
[42] George, JM., Jin, H., Hoods, WS. and Clayton, DF. Characterization of a novel protein regulated during the critical period for song learning in the zebra finch. Neuron 15: 361-372, 1995.
[43] Gharib, A., Sarda, N., Chabannes, B., Cronenberger, L. and Pacheco, H. The regional concentrations of S-adenosyl-L-homocysteine and adenosine in rat brain. J. Neurochem. 38: 810-815, 1982.
[44] Giasson, BI. and Mushynski, WE. Aberrant stress-induced phosphorylation of perikaryal neurofilaments. J. Biol. Chem. 271: 30404- 30409, 1990.
[45] Giasson, BI., Galvin, JE., Lee, VM. and Trojanowski JQ. The cellular and molecular pathology of Parkinson disease. In: *Neurodegenerative Dementias, Eds:* Clark, CM. and Trojanowski, JQ, McGraw-Hill, New York, Cpt 16: 219-228, 2000.
[46] Greenfield, JG. and Bosanquet, FD. The brainstem lesions in Parkinsonism. J. Neurol Neurosurg Psychiat 16: 213-126, 1953.
[47] Guggenheim, M.A., Couch, JR. and Weinberg, W. Motor dysfunction as a permanent complication of methanol ingestion. Presentation of a case with a beneficial response to levodopa treatment. Arch. Neurol. 24: 550-554, 1971.
[48] Hayes, M., Porter, JA., Chiang, C., Chang, D., Tessier-Lavigne, M., Beachy, PA. and Rosenthal, A. Induction of midbrain dopaminergic neurons by Sonic hedgehog. Neuron 15: 35-44, 1995.
[49] Hirata, F. and Axelrod, J. Phospholipid methylation and biological signal transmission. Science 209: 1082-1089, 1980.
[50] Hochberg, F., Miller, G., Valenzuela, R., et al: Late motor defecits of Chilean manganese miners: a blinded control study. Neurology 47: 788-795, 1996.
[51] Hornykiewicz, O. Dopamine (3-hydroxytryamine) and function. Pharmacol Rev 18: 925-964, 1966.
[52] Ince, PG and Codd, GA. Return of the cycad hypothesis-does the amyotrophic lateral sclerosis/parkinsonism dementia complex (ALS/PDC) of Guam have new implications for global health? Neuropathol. Appl. Neurobiol. 31: 345-353, 2005.
[53] Iwatsubo, T., Nakano, I., Fugunaga, K. and Miyamoto, E. Ca2+/calmodulin-dependent protein kinase II immunoreactivity in Lewy's bodies. Acta Neuropathol. 82: 159-163, 1991.
[54] Jager, DH and Bethlem, JJ. The distribution of Lewy bodies in the central and autonomic nervous systems in idiopathic paralysis agitans. Neurol. Neurosurg. Psychiat. 23: 283-290 1960.
[55] Jager, WA. Den Sphingomyelin in Lewy includes bodies in Parkinson's disease. Arch. Neurol. (Chicago) 21: 615-619, 1969.
[56] Julien, JP. and Muskynaki, WE. Multiple phosphorylation sites in mammalian neuro-filamant polypeptides. J. Biol. Chem. 257: 10467-10470, 1998.

[57] Kitada, T,, Asakawa, S., Hattori, N., Matsumine, H., Yamamura, Y., Minoshima, S., Yokochi, M., Mizono, Y. and Shimizu, N. Mutations in the parkin gene cause autosomal recessive juvenile parkinsonism. Nature 392 (6676): 605-608, 1998.
[58] Koller, WC. And Huber, SJ. Tremor disorders of aging: Diagnosis and management. Geriatrics 44: 33-36, 1989.
[59] Kosel, S., Lucking, CB., Egensperger, R., Mehraein, P. and Graeber, MB. Mitochondrial NADH dehydrogenase and CYP2D genotypes in Lewy-body parkinsonism. J. Neurosci. Res. 44(2): 174-183, 1996.
[60] Kotb, M. and Geller, AM. Methionine adenosyltransferase: Structure and function. Pharm. Therap. 59(2(: 125-143, 1993
[61] Kruger, R., Vieir-Saecker, AM, Khun, W. et al. Increased susceptibility in sparadic Parkinson's disease by certain combined alpha-synuclein/apolipoprotein E genotype. Ann. Neurol 45: 611-617, 1999.
[62] Kruger, S., Kuhn, WT., Woitalla, D. et al. Ala30Pro mutation in the gene encoding alpha-synuclein in Parkinson disease. Nat. Genet 18: 106-108, 1998.
[63] Kuhn, W., Muller, T., Grosse, H. and Rommelspacher, H. Elevated levels of Harman and norharman in cerebrospinal fluid of Parkinson's disease patients. J. Neural Transm. 103: 1435-1440, 1996.
[64] Langston, JW. And Forno, LS. The hypothalamus in Parkinson's disease. Ann. Neurol. 3: 129-133, 1978.
[65] Lansbury, PT. and Brice, A. Genetics of Parkinson's disease and biochemical studies of implicated gene products. Curr. Opin. Cell Biol. 14: 653-660, 2002.
[66] Lee, V., Carden, ML., Schlaepfer, WW., Trojanowski, JQ. Monoclonal antibodies distinguish several differently phosphorylated states of the two largest rat neurofilament subunits (NF-H and NF-M) and demonstrate their existence in the normal nervous system of adult rats. J. Neurosci. 7: 3474-3488, 1987.
[67] Lee, E. and Charlton, C. One-methyl-4-phenylpyridinium (MPP^+) increases S-adenosyl-methionine dependent phospholipid methylation. Pharm. Biochem. and Beh. 70: 105-114, 2001.
[68] Lee, EY., Chen, H., Shepherd, KR., Lamango, NS., Soliman, KF. and Charlton, CG. The inhibitory role of methylation on the binding characteristics of dopamine receptors and transporter. Neurosci. Res. 48: 335-344, 2004.
[69] Lee, ES., Chen, H., Hardman, H., Simm, A and Charlton, C. Excessive S-adenosyl.L-methionine-dependent methylation increases levels of methanol, formaldehyde and formic acid in rat brain striatal homogenate: Possible role in S-adenosyl-L-methionie–induced Parkinson's disease-like disorders. Life Sci. 3: 821-827, 2008.
[70] Lee, ES., Chen, H., Soliman, KF. and Charlton, CG. Effects of homocysteine on the dopaminergic system and behavior in rodents. NeuroToxicology 26 (3): 361-371, 2005.
[71] Lee, ES., Chen, H., Shepherd, K., Lamango, NS, Soliman, KF. and Charlton, CG. The inhibitory role of methylation on the binding characteristics of dopamine receptors and transporter. Neurosci. Res. 48: 335-244, 2004.
[72] Lee, ES., Soliman, KF and Charlton, CG. Lyso-phosphatidylcholine decreases locomotor activities and dopamine turnover rate in rats. NeuroToxicol 26: 27-38, 2005.

[73] Lee, FJ., Choi, C. and Lee, SJ. Membrane bound alpha-synuclein has a high aggregation propensity and the ability to seed the aggregation of the cytosolic form. J. Biol. Chem. 277: 671-678, 2002.

[74] Lee, FJ., Liu, F., Pristupa, ZB. and Niznik, HB. Direct binding and functional coupling of alpha-synuclein to the dopamine transporters accelerate dopamine-induced apoptosis. FASEB J. 15: 916-926, 2001.

[75] Lee, ES. and Charlton, C. One-methyl-4-phenylpyridinium (MPP+) increases S-adenosylmethionine-dependent phospholipid methylation. Pharmacol. Biochem. Beh. 70: 105-114, 2001.

[76] Leroy, E., Anastosooulos, D., Konitsiotis, S., Larken, C. and Polymeropoulos, MN. Deletions in the Parkin gene and genetic heterogencity in a Greek family with earcy onset Parkinson disease. Hum. Genet. 103(4): 424-427. 1998.

[77] Levitan, IB. and Kaczmarek, LK. The birth and death of a neuron. In: *The Neuron: Cell and Molecular Biology*. 3rd ed, pp. 375-393. 2002.

[78] Ma, SY., Roytta, M., Rinne, JO., Collan, Y. and Rinne, UK. Correlation between neuromorphometry in the substantia nigra and clinical features in Parkinson's disease using dissector counts. J. Neurol. Scs. 151: 83-87, 1997.

[79] Mann, SP. and Hill, MW. Activation and inactivation of striatal tyrosine hydroxylase: the effects of pH, ATP and cyclic AMP, S-adenosylmethionine and S-adenosylhomocysteine Biochem. Pharmacology 32: 3369-3374, 1983.

[80] Matsubara, K., Aoyama, K., Suma, M. and Awaya, T. N-methylation underlying Parkinson's disease. Neurotoxicology and Teratology 24: 593-598, 2002.

[81] Mays, LI., Borek, E. and Finch, CE. Glycine N-methyltransferase is a regulatory enzyme which increases in aging animals. Nature 243, 411-413, 1973.

[82] McGeer, PL. and Steele, JC. The ALS/PDC syndrome of Guam: Potential biomarkers for an enigmatic disorder. Prog. Neurobio. 95: 663-669, 2011.

[83] Murray, MP., Kory, RC. and Clarkson, BH. Walking patterns in healthy old men. J. Gerontol. 24: 169-178, 1969.

[84] Muruyama, W., Abe, T., Tohgi, H., Dostert, P. and Naoi, M. A dopaminergic neurotoxin, (R)-N-methylsalsolinol increases in parkinsonism cerebrospinal fluid. Ann. Neurol. 40: 119-112, 1996.

[85] Muthian, G., Mackey, V., King, J. and Charlton, C. Modeling a Sensitization stage and a Precipitation stage for Parkinson's disease using Prenatal and Postnatal 1-Methyl-4-phenyl-1,2,3,4-tetrahydropyridine (MPTP) administration. Neurosci. J. 169: 1085-1093, 2010.

[86] Nagatsu, T. and Yoshida, M. An endogenous substance of the brain, terrahydroisoquinoline, produces parkinsonism in primates with decreased dopamine, tyrosine hydroxylase and biopterin in the nigrostriatal regions. Neurosci. Lett. 87: 178-182, 1988.

[87] Nakamura, S., Kawamoto, Y., Nakano, S. et al. p35nck5a and cyclin-dependent kinase 5 colocalize in Lewy bodies of brains with Parkinson's disease. Acta Neuropathol. 94: 153- 157, 1997.

[88] Naoi, M., Maruyama, W., Yukihiro, A. and Yi, H. Dopamine-derived endogenous N-methyl-(R)-salsolinol. Its role in Parkinson's disease. Neurotoxi. and Teratol. 24: 579-591, 2002.

[89] Ochi, N., Naoi, M., Mogi, M., Ohya, Y., Mizutani, N., Watanabe, K., Harada, M. and Hagatsu, T. Effects of 1-methyl-4-phenyl-1,2,3,6-tetrahydropyridine (MPTP) administration in prenatal stage on the dopamine system in the postnatal mouse brain. Life Sci. 48(3): 217-223, 1991.

[90] Ohama, E. and Ikuta, F. Parkinson disease distribution of Lewy bodies and monoamine neuron system. Acta Neuropathol. (Berl) 34: 311-319, 1976.

[91] Oppenheim, RW. Cell death during development of the nervous system. Annu. Rev. Neurosci. 14: 453–501, 1991.

[92] Ortel, WH., Bandmann, O., Eichhorn, T. and Glasser, T. Peripheral markers of PD. An overview. In: *Neurology*, vol 69, Ed: Battistin, L., Scarlato, G., Caraceni, T. and Ruggieri, S. Lippincott-Raven Publishers, Philadelphia, pp 283-291,1996.

[93] Oyanagi, K. The nature of the parkinsonian-dementia complex and amyotrophic lateral sclerosis of Guam and magnesium deficiency. Parkinsonism and Related Disorders 11: S17-S23, 2005.

[94] Papadimitrior, A., Veleta, V., Hadjigerogiou, GM. et al. Mutated alpha-synuclein gene in two Greek kindreds with familial PD: incomplete penetrance. Neurology 52:651-564, 1999.

[95] Perrone-Capano, C and di Porzio, U. Epigenetic factors and midbrain dopaminergic neurone development. BioEssays 18 (10): 817-824, 1996.

[96] Pollanen, MS., Dicken, DW., Bergeron, C. Pathology and biology of Lewy's body. J. Neuropathol. Exp. Neurol. 52: 183-191, 1993.

[97] Polymeropoulos, MN., Lavedan, C., Leroy, E. et al. Mutations in alpha-synuclein gene identified in families with Parkinson disease. Science 276:2045-2047, 1997.

[98] Rajput, AH. and Rozdilsky, B. Dysautonomia in parkinsonism: a clinicopathological study. J. Jeurol. Neurosurg. Psychiatr. 39: 1092-1100, 1970.

[99] Ravenholt RT. Influeza, Encephalitis Lethargica, Parkinsonism. Lancet 326 (8303): 860-864, 1982.

[100] Ren, Y., Zhao, J. and Feng J. Parkin binds to alpha and beta tubulin and increases their ubiquitination and degradation. J. Neurosci. 23 (8): 3316-3324, 2003.

[101] Sabbagh, N., Bruce, A., Marez, D., Durr, A., Legrand, M., Loguidice, JM., Destce, A., Agrid, Y. and Broly, F. CYP2D6 polymorphism and Parkinson disease susceptibility. Mov. Disord. 14: 230-236, 1999.

[102] Sacks, O. Cycad island. In: The Island of the Colorblind. New York: Vintage, pp 97-177, 1998.

[103] Schneider, JS., Yuwiler, A. and Markham, CH. Production of Parkinson-like syndrome in the cat with N- methyl-4- phenyl-1,2,3,6- trtrahydropyridine. Proc. Natl. Acad. Sci. USA. 80: 293-307, 1983.

[104] Selby, G. Cerebral atrophy in parkinsonism. J. Neurol. Sci. 6: 517-559, 1968.

[105] Sellinger, OZ., Kramer, CM., Conger, A. and Duboff, GS. The carboxylmethylation of cerebral membrane-bound proteins increases with age. Mechanisms of Aging and Develop 43: 161-173,1988.

[106] Schwartz, JH. Synthesis and trafficking of neural proteins. In: Principles of Neural Science. 3rd ed. Eds: Kandal, ER., Schwartz, JH. And Jessel, TM. Appleton and Lange, Norwalk, pp 49-65, 1991.

[107] Solomon, MJ., Larsen, P. and Varshavsky, A. Mapping protein-DNA interactions in vivo with formaldehyde: evidence that histone H4 is retained on a highly transcribed gene. Cell 53: 937-947, 1988.

[108] Spencer, PS., Nunn, P., Hugon, J., Ludolph, A. and Roy, DN. Motorneurone disease on Guam: Possible role of food neurotoxin. Lancet 327 (8487, 965, 1986.

[109] Spenser, P. Guam ALS/parkinsonism-dementia: a long-latency neurotoxic disorder caused by a "slow" toxin(s) in food. Can J. Neurol. Sci 14: 347-357, 1987.

[110] Spillantini, MG., Schmidt, ML., Lee, VMY., et al. Alpha-synuclein in Lewy's bodies. Nature 388: 839-840, 1997.

[111] Sternberger, LA. and Sternberger, NH. Monoclonal antibodies distinguish phosphorylated and nonphosphorylated forms of neurofilaments in situ. Proc. Natl. Acad. Sci. USA. 80: 6126-6130, 1983.

[112] Stramentinoli, G., Gualano, M., Catto, E. and Algeri, S. Tissue levels of S-adenosyl-methionine in aging rats. J. Gerontol. 32(4): 392-394, 1977.

[113] Tarlaci, S. Vincristine-induced fetal neuropathy in non-Hodkin's lymphoma. Neurotoxicol. 29 (4): 748-749, 2008.

[114] Tretiakoff, C. Contribution a l'etude de l'anatomic pathologique du locus niger de Soemmering avec quelique deductions relatives a la pathogenia des troubles du tonus musculaire de la maladie de Parkinson. Thesis. Paris. (1919). Cited in Schultz, Prog. Neurol. 18:12-166. 1982.

[115] van Duinen, SG., Lammers, GL., Matt-Schieman, MLC. And Roos, RAC. Numerous and widespread alpha synuclein-negative Lewy's bodies in an asymptomatic patient. Acta Neuropathol. 97: 533-539, 1999.

[116] Vanderhaegen, JJ., Poirior, O. and Steronon, JE. Pathological findings in idiopathic orthostatic hypotension. Arch. Neurol. 11:207-214, 1970.

[117] Voorn, P., Kalsbeek, A., Jorritsma-Byham, B. and Groenewa-jen, HJ. The pre- and post-natal development of the dopaminergic cell groups in the ventral mesencephalon and the dopaminergic innervation of the striat irn of the rat. Neuroscience 25: 857-887, 1988.

[118] Waite, LM., Broe, GA., Creasey, H. et al. Neurological signs, aging and neurodegenerative syndromes. Arch. Neurol. 53: 498-502, 1996.

[119] Ward, CD., Duvosin, RC., Ince, SE., Nutt, JD. and Calne, DB. Parkinson's disease in 65 pairs of twins and in a set of quadruplets. Neurology 33: 815-824, 1983.

[120] Weiss, AD. The locus of reaction time change with set, motivation and age. J. Gerontol. 20: 60-64, 1965.

[121] Welford, AT. Motor performance. In: *Handbook of the Psychology of Aging*. Eds: Birren, JE. And Schaine, KW, New York, Van Nostrand Reinhold, pp 450-496, 1977.

[122] Wesemann, W., Grote, C., Clement, HW., Block, F. and Sontag, KH. Functional studies on monoaminergic transmitter release in parkinosonism. Prog. Neuropsychopharmacol. Biol. Psychiatry 17: 487-499, 1993.

[123] Williams, AC. and Ramsden, DB. Nicotinamide homeostasis: A xenobiotic pathway that is key to development and degenerative diseases. Medical Hypothesis 65: 353-362, 2005.

[124] Williams, AC., Pall, HS., Steventon, GB., Green, S., Buttrum, S.,Molly, H. and Waring, RR. N-methylation of pyridines and Parkinson's disease. Adv. Neurol. 60: 194-196, 1993.

[125] Withers, GS., George, JM., Banker, GA. and Clayton, DF. Delayed localization of synelfin (synuclein, NACP) to presynaptic terminals in cultured rat hippocampal neurons Dev. Brain Res. 99: 87-94, 1997.

[126] Yahr, MD. and Bering, EA. In: Parkinson disease. Present status and research trends. Eds. Yahr MD and Dering, EA. US-DHEW PP47. 1968.

[127] Zhoa, W., Latinwo, L., Liu, XX., Lee, E., Lamango, N. and Charlton, C. L-dopa upregulates the expression and activities of methionine adenosyl transferase and catechol-O-methyltransferase. Exprl. Neurology. 171, 127-138, 2001.

Basal Ganglia and the Error Monitoring and Processing System: How Alcohol Modulates the Error Monitoring and Processing Capacity of the Basal Ganglia

M.O. Welcome and V.A. Pereverzev

Additional information is available at the end of the chapter

http://dx.doi.org/10.5772/53945

1. Introduction

The Basal ganglia as a subcortical relay station at the base of the forebrain is largely involved in processing of information, cognition, and movement (Gehring et al. 1993; Mathalon et al., 2003; Nick et al., 2003). Over the last century, knowledge about the basal ganglia has been acquired mainly from animal research, and pathologies that affect the basal ganglia in humans. In pathologies such as Parkinson's and Huntington's' diseases the basal ganglia's functions are greatly affected (Beste et al., 2009; Holroyd et al., 2002).

Apart from brain pathologies, psychotic substances can affect the normal functioning of the basal ganglia (Goldstein et al., 2007). Alcohol is one of the psychotic substances that affect the functions of the basal ganglia (Goldstein et al., 2007; Holroyd & Yeung 2003; Goodlett & Horn 2001).

Many substances that cross the blood brain barrier can affect the normal functioning of the basal ganglia either indirectly or directly (Buhler et al., 1983). The direct effect occurs, if the substances reach the basal nuclei. The indirect effect happens when pathways linking other brain regions (sub-cortical pathways) are affected. In addition, the metabolic products of these substances can exert their effect on the neurons of the basal ganglia or on the pathways linking the basal ganglia (Buhler et al., 1983; Deitrich et al 2006; Salvador & Alfredo 2010).

In recent years, the basal ganglia have been implicated in error commission (Holroyd & Yeung 2003). In fact, in pathologies involving the basal ganglia, research has shown that error commission rate is significantly higher, compared to controls (Holroyd et al., 2002).

In this chapter, we examined the effect of alcohol on the functions (precisely the error monitoring and processing capacity) of the basal ganglia.

2. Materials and methods

Literatures for this study were searched in Pubmed, DOAJ, Embase, Google scholar, African Online Journals, and Scopus. The following keywords were used in the search processes: Alcohol and error detection; Alcohol and correction; Alcohol and error commission; Alcohol and error processing (OR monitoring); error monitoring and processing system; basal ganglia; error and the basal ganglia; alcohol and the basal ganglia. For details on the study materials and methods, see Welcome et al., 2010. In addition, we analyzed our recent data as regards to error commission dynamics in alcohol users and non-alcohol users. Data from our recent publications regarding error commission and effectiveness of cognitive functions in alcohol users and non-alcohol users were also examined.

3. Basal ganglia and the error monitoring and processing system

The error monitoring and processing system (EMPS) located in the substantia nigra of the midbrain, basal ganglia and cortex of the forebrain, plays a leading role in error detection and correction. Although, it is widely known that the main components of EMPS are the dopaminergic system and anterior cingulate cortex, it appears that the basal ganglia also play a crucial role (Welcome et al., 2010).

Recent data suggest that error commission is tightly monitored by the basal ganglia, and this anatomical structure remains an integral aspect of cognitive processing (Beste et al., 2009; Holroyd & Coles 2002). Importantly, an increase in error commission is associated with decrease in cognitive functions (Welcome et al., 2010, 2011). The basal ganglia are adequately engaged with other brain areas and monitors error detection and correction (Carter et al., 1999; Garavan et al., 2002; Holroyd & Yeung 2003). The functions of the EMPS are dependent on the degree of phasic dopamine activity on the brain areas that process and monitor error commission (Holroyd & Yeung 2003). Other neuromediators (GABA, glycine) might also play crucial role (Wick et al., 1998).

3.1. Error commission: Different types, one source

Daily performances of humans are in most cases evaluated based on the outcome of activities executed. The activity function is a measure of accuracy of performance (i.e. speed of performance and the number of incorrect/correct tasks done). While the speed of tasks might be controversial in some cases, error commission rate remains a useful parameter in performance evaluation. For instance, in basal ganglia pathologies, error commission has been found to significantly increase, whereas speed of task decreases. On the contrary, even though error commission might increase in alcohol users, our data and those of other authors show faster performance of tasks in this group of people (Welcome et al., 2010; Schulte et al., 2001).

The results of our research further stipulate that a normal physiological error commission rate by humans who do not use alcohol is approximately 5%, whereas the rate for alcohol users significantly exceeds 10% (Welcome et al., 2010). This is because the brain processing of information has an automatic component, which means a basal level of error commission for a normal physiological state. Lower error commission points to more effective processing in those brain regions responsible for correct responses. Correct responses tightly engaged a network comprising the left lateral prefrontal cortex, left postcentral gyrus/inferior parietal lobule, striatum, and left cerebellum (Garavan et al., 2002; Marco-Pallarés et al., 2008; Endrass et al., 2012).

The evolution of error processing is a complex one. In comparative evolutionary studies, there are evidences that suggest intrinsic error processes not only at the organismal level, but also at the cellular and subcellular level (cellular and genetic errors) (Schulte et al., 2001; Ochoa 2006; Takeuchi et al., 2005; Cohen & Ellwein 1991). Increased error commission seen in the real world (organismal level of error commission) is the result of error processing disorder at the neuronal level (Holroyd & Coles 2002). It is important to note that many catastrophic cases (in aviation, for instance) are caused by error commission – a failure in the brain's error monitoring and processing function or the so-called "human factor". Further study in this aspect will be of great importance to enhance safety and increase effectiveness of mental performance, especially for the necessary contingents of people such as pilots.

There are different types of errors, but almost all types have one source – the EMPS. In experimental conditions, errors are made when subject press the incorrect button on a keyboard (for example, in a Go/No-Go task) or did not pick the correct answer, or adhere strictly to instructions (Stevens et al., 2009). These errors are further classified by some authors as memory commission/omission errors; brain errors; cognitive errors etc. – all from one source – the EMPS (Giesbrecht et al., 2007; Hurst 2008; Stevens et al., 2009). Error of omission occurs as a failure to respond to tasks. The electrophysiological bases of these two types of errors are outlined in a recent work by Krigolson & Holroyd (2007). Errors committed in the medical setting (by medics) have been referred to as medical errors – which are cognitive errors of omission or commission (for review see Hurst 2008).

Another important question that comes into mind is – how do we know an error is made? Firstly, in an experimental condition, a deviation from the set goals will be decoded as error. However, in certain cases, even the participants recognize the fact that they committed error. So how does this happen? A search for the answer to this question is rooted in the less researched Pe component following ERN (Pe component is briefly discussed below). Research suggests that behavioral adjustment might represent a useful in error awareness. There evidences suggest a close relationship among error commission, behavioral adjustment and executive functions (Garavan et al., 2002; Marco-Pallarés et al., 2008). The awareness of errors might be the result of close engagement between executive functions and the brain EMPS. Hence, it is probable that when executive functions (e.g. attention) are closely engaged with the EMPS, error awareness increases. Furthermore, recent evidence shows the capacity of the basal ganglia (through the basal ganglia-cortical pathways) to implement successful performances that were initially produced by other brain regions, indicating precise functional connections between basal ganglia circuits and the motor regions that directly control performance (Charlesworth et al., 2012). Also, the basal ganglia generate a variety of behaviors during execution of task and learn to implement the successful behaviors in their repertoire to meet the target (Sur & Schultz 1999).

In electrophysiological studies, error commission is reflected in the reduced amplitude of the Error Related Negativity, ERN (or Error Negativity, Ne) (Falkenstein et al., 2000; Ridderinkhof et al., 2002), a negative deflection in the electroencephalogram with a maximum in the midline of the frontocentral region of the scalp having a latent period around 50-150ms (Falkenstein et al., 2000; Ridderinkhof et al., 2002).

The ERN amplitude might show gradual decrease for older adults (Pontifex et al., 2010). However, because of amplitude difference across different age groups caused by gradual increase in brain regions involved in error processing, the number of brain regions responsible for error processing and monitoring may vary according to the age of the subjects under analysis. Importantly, not only maturation of the neural systems that identifies different errors account for this increase (Stevens et al., 2009), but also neural plasticity. ERN is smaller for adolescents (Pontifex et al., 2010).

Nowadays, a growing body of data suggests that error commission is associated not only with the early time-course ERN components of the electroencephalogram but also with a successive neurophysiological late error positivity (Pe) following motor execution. The exact cognitive and physiological processes contributing to these two components, as well as their functional independence, are still not fully been unraveled (Vocat et al., 2008). The occurrences of ERN and Pe involve activation of a distinct configuration of intracranial generators during error commission. Pe peaks approximately at approximately 300ms after erroneous actions (Vocat et al., 2008; Endrass et al., 2012).

For about two decades the Pe component has remained elusive and has become the subject of a fierce debate in the scientific community (Falkenstein et al., 2000; Vocat et al., 2008; Dhar M et al., 2011).

Several studies have suggested that the error positivity (Pe) reflect conscious error awareness (Dhar et al. 2011; Garavan et al., 2002; Marco-Pallarés et al., 2008). Although, previous studies have disputed this view. According to Falkenstein *et al.* (2000) the Pe, represent a error-specific component, which is independent of the ERN, and hence is associated with a later aspect of error processing or post-error processing. Falkenstein and coauthors (2000) further argue that the Pe reflects conscious error processing or the post-error adjustment of response strategies.

A recent report further supports the error awareness property of the Pe component. Endrass and colleagues (2012) have recently shown that error awareness mainly influences the Pe, whereas the ERN seems unaffected by conscious awareness of an error. This confirms that the Pe is related to error commission. Hence this component is sensitive to the salience of an error and that salience secondarily may trigger error awareness (for review see Endrass et al., 2012).

For review on ERN and Pe amplitude see Amodio *et al.* (2006), Endrass *et al.* (2012), Pontifex *et al.* (2010), Falkenstein *et al.* (2000).

3.2. Error commission in controls, and Basal ganglia pathologies

Because both ERN and Pe show promise for use in clinical setting for the diagnosis of psychopathology (including basal ganglia pathologies), further research on these components is necessary. To this end, reports clearly indicate that these error components may represent a predisposition factor for behavioral disorders including substance use disorders (alcoholism), brain (basal ganglia) pathologies (Olvet & Hajcak 2008; Franken et al., 2010; Fein & Chang 2008; Van Veen & Carter 2006; Aarts & Pourtois 2010). Although, there are controversies on whether or not the ERN actually has a diagnostic significance. Studies have suggested that the ERN reflect a trait, and not a state factor (Pailing & Segalowitz 2004; Olvet & Hajcak 2008). For a better appreciation of the usefulness of ERN and Pe in psychopathology (including basal ganglia dysfunctions) a mathematical modeling involving the second derivative of these components and segmental analysis might be necessary which will give a glimpse into their importance for clinical diagnosis.

Besides alcohol and basal ganglia pathologies, sleep deprivation (or insomnia) is also a factor for increase in error commission which might result in various catastrophes including industrial and engineering disasters, motor accidents etc. (Mitler et al., 1988). This suggests the presence of a circadian control mechanism in EMPS.

Vocat *et al.* (2008) found that the ERN correlates with the level of state anxiety, even in the subclinical range, whereas the Pe correlates negatively with the total number of errors and positively with the improvement of response speed on correct trials.

The mechanism of increase in error commission in people with basal ganglia dysfunction is a complex one. A growing body of literature data suggests the involvement of attention control mechanisms. For instance, patients with Huntington's disease show great decrease in the ability to assess various aspects of tasks (disorder in attention), resulting from a disorder in action-selection processes. This obviously will lead to increase in error commission in tasks (Beste et al., 2008). One recent study by Bocquillon and co-workers (2012) suggests that basal ganglia pathologies results in resistance impairment to distracters (which might actually, in most cases represent competing neural information), hence providing more grounds for error commission. An electromagnetic tomography and electrophysiological study involving the P300 found that, unlike in the controls, in patients with Parkinson's disease, disruption of the frontoparietal network impaired resistance to distracters, which resulted in attention disorders (Bocquillon et al., 2012). However, increase in error commission may in part be the result of global cognitive impairment and inhibitory control disorders (Gauggel et al., 2004).

In another study, Beste *et al.* (2006) assessed ERN amplitude in a speeded reaction task under consideration of the underlying genetic abnormalities in patients with Huntington's disease. The findings of the researchers showed a specific reduction in the ERN, suggesting impaired error processing. Furthermore, the ERN was closely related to the trinucleotide

CAG-repeat expansion. The authors concluded that the reduction of the ERN is likely to be an effect of the dopaminergic pathology. And that the ERN might be a measure for the integrity of striatal dopaminergic output function (Beste et al., 2006). This view is in direct agreement with previous studies on the role of the dopaminergic system in error commission (Holroyd & Yeung 2003). In contrary to the study of Beste and colleagues (2006), previous study by Holroyd and colleagues (2002) did not find any difference in ERN amplitude between patients with basal ganglia pathology (precisely Parkinson disease) and the controls. Although the authors noted that the error-processing system associated with the ERN was not severely compromised in the patient population that participated in the study.

Patients with basal ganglia pathologies have slower reaction time compared to controls (Berry et al., 1999). It appears that time processing disorders might even be a more useful factor to assess basal ganglia pathologies (Beste et al., 2007). In a time-estimation and time-discrimination task Beste *et al.* (2007) found deterioration of time-estimation processes in symptomatic and even presymptomatic Huntington's disease. However, time-discrimination processes were not affected. Time processing is a critical function of the cortico-basal ganglia circuits (Jin et al., 2009). Although previous report has disputed the involvement of the basal ganglia in timing (Aparicio et al., 2005). A general probation of the components of error processing in various cultural groups, while controlling for factors such as age, gender, educational level, various mental states, and psychopathologies is necessary.

4. Pathways of alcohol's action on the error monitoring and processing capacity of the Basal ganglia

For the first time in 2002, it was reported that alcohol consumption disrupts error monitoring (Ridderinkhof et al., 2002). According to electro-physiological studies, the effect of alcohol on the Error Monitoring and Processing System, EMPS is reflected in the reduced amplitude of the Error Related Negativity (ERN) (Falkenstein et al., 1995; Ridderinkhof et al., 2002), a negative deflection in the electroencephalogram with a maximum in the midline of the frontocentral region of the scalp having a latent period around 50-150ms (Easdon et al., 2005; Ridderinkhof et al., 2002; Welcome et al., 2010).

Even though the effect of alcohol on EMPS is documented, information on how alcohol affects error monitoring and processing is scanty (i.e. the mechanism of alcohol's effect on EMPS remain adequately researched). Two co-researchers, Holroyd and Yeung in 2003 in their review suggested that alcohol's effect on error monitoring and processing is likely indirect, not direct, and that the mechanisms remained unknown. They however suggested that alcohol might modulate EMPS through its effect on the dopamine system. Recently, in our review we suggested indirect mechanisms by which alcohol disrupts the EMPS (Welcome et al., 2010). However, based on increasing evidences (Deitrich et al., 2006; Wick et al., 1998; Quertemont 2004; Buhler et al., 1983), a direct disruption might also be possible, especially, if we consider the possibility that receptors of neuromediators might have "alcohol pockets-receptors". It is reported that glycine and $GABA_A$ receptors may harbor specific pockets for alcohol (Wick et al., 1998).

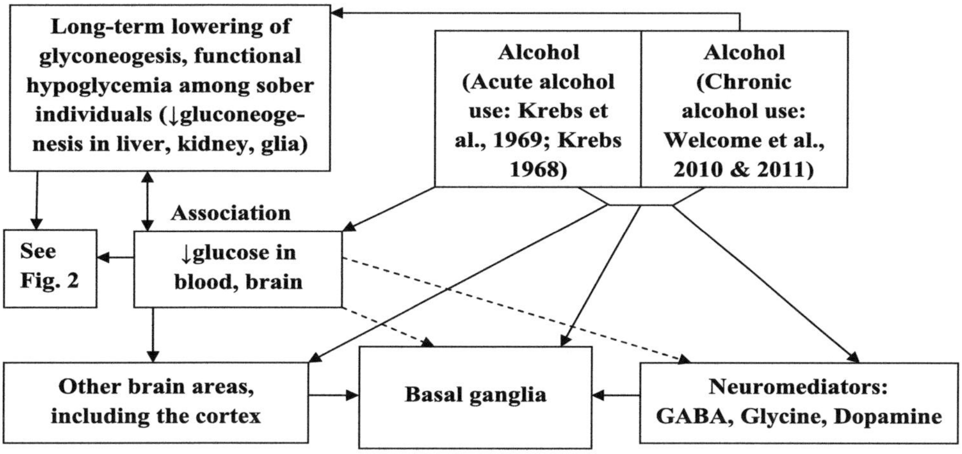

Figure 1. Pathways of alcohol's action on the Basal Ganglia

Besides, it is known that alcohol readily crosses the blood brain barrier. In the brain, alcohol can disrupt the transmission of signals through the basal ganglia/or the processing of information by the basal ganglia. The following scenarios are possible (see fig. 1):

a. Direct effect of alcohol on the processing capacity of the basal ganglia by inhibiting cellular processes, depending on the dose of alcohol;
b. Indirect effect of alcohol on the processing capacity of the basal ganglia by affecting other brain areas connected to the basal ganglia;
c. Direct effect on neuromediators that modulate the processing of information in the basal ganglia and/or associated brain pathways;
d. Action of alcohol metabolites (acetaldehyde; acetate; protein, lipid, enzyme & DNA adducts of alcohol) on the processing of information in the basal ganglia and/or associated brain pathways. The brain might contain alcohol metabolizing enzymes such as ADH-1, ADH-2, ADH-3 (might play little or no role), CYP P4502E1 (Quertemont 2004; Buhler et al., 1983), although there might be a huge genetic variance. It important to note that injection of acetate into the brain causes significant decrease in motor function (Deitrich et al., 2006).

5. Theories suggesting alcohol's effect on the error monitoring and processing capacity of the Basal ganglia

There are at least five hypotheses & theories that might explain how alcohol use affects the error monitoring and processing capacity of the basal ganglia. They are hypotheses of error detection; reinforcement-learning theory; conflict-monitoring theory; the integrated conflict monitoring-reinforcement learning theory; and hypothesis of alcohol-related glucose-dependent system of error monitoring & processing (Holroyd & Coles 2002; Holroyd &

Yeung 2003; Welcome et al., 2010). Of these theories/hypotheses, only the reinforcement-learning theory; conflict-monitoring theory; and the integrated conflict monitoring-reinforcement learning theory is close to defining the role of basal ganglia in the EMPS. The hypothesis of alcohol-related glucose-dependent system of error monitoring & processing (ARGD-EMPS Hypothesis) suggests a mechanism of alcohol's effect on the EMPS (Welcome et al., 2010).

5.1. The reinforcement learning theory

One of the integral properties of the basal ganglia is to determine whether the end-result of events will be favorable or not; and is crucial to the functioning of EMPS. The basal ganglia monitor and steadily predict the result of ongoing events (Welcome et al., 2010; Botvinick et al., 2001 & 2004; Holroyd & Yeung 2003; Garavan et al., 2002; Gehring et al., 1993 & 2001). The basal ganglia is one of the many brain structures that send command information to the ACC for further processing (it is presently not clear the kind of information that might require further processing in ACC, or whether these processes only represent one of the many brain mechanisms for safety) (Holroyd & Coles 2002; Holroyd & Yeung 2003; Welcome et al., 2010). It is however, possible that these command information are too complex for only the basal ganglia to process, hence need other more specialized locations. That is why the ACC functions as a selector for conflicted command. This is why the ACC is regarded as a control filter (Welcome et al., 2010; Carter et al., 1998; Nieuwenhuis et al., 2003; Ridderinkhof et al., 2003). The major neuromediator here is dopamine. Its tonic activity depends on reinforcing properties of alcohol (Holroyd & Yeung 2003; Munte et al., 2008; Montague et al., 1996). Alcohol may increase the tonic activity of dopamine system and subsequently leading to inhibition of neuronal activity, the result is increased error commission (Welcome et al., 2010; Holroyd & Yeung 2003; Easdon et al., 2005).

5.2. The conflict-monitoring theory

Although there are less information as regards to this theory with respect to the basal ganglia. Research suggests that the basal ganglia may be actively engaged with other systems to monitor conflict (through the sub-cortical pathways). This is an important aspect of information processing for cognitive control (Botvinick et al., 2001 & 2004; Welcome et al., 2010; Gehring et al., 2001). Conflict occurs as a result of simultaneous activation of different regions, controlling the activation of different levels of competing motor control units in the motor cortex. Processing of stimulus is characterized by constant flow of activity in the pathways that send stimulus related information to the cortex of the hindbrain, and subsequently results in the corresponding response in the motor cortex (Botvinick et al., 2001 & 2004; Welcome et al., 2010). Distractive stimulus may activate incorrect response in this system (Goldstein et al., 2007; Holroyd & Coles 2002). Alcohol related disruption of information processing decreases the activation of correct responses (through its inhibitory effect) (Holroyd & Yeung 2003). In addition to the dopamine system (Holroyd & Coles 2002), GABA and glycine might also play a role (Wick et al., 1998).

5.3. Integrated conflict monitoring-reinforcement learning theory

In view of this theory, although not fully clear, the basal ganglia generate error signals (i.e. the basal ganglia undertake processing of input signals, and are end-result predictors). Hence, the basal ganglia have been referred to as adaptive critics. It is also possible that the error signals processed in the basal ganglia are received from ACC (Ridderinkhof et al., 2003; Umhau et al., 2003). Sometimes, however, end-result can be different from the input signal (especially when result was not predicted). The resultant effect is a shift in dopamine signal. The error produced is called temporal difference error. These errors are sent through the dopamine system to other brain regions for further analysis: a) motor control systems (such as dorsolateral prefrontal cortex, amygdala); b) control filter (ACC); c) and again to the basal ganglia. These processes suggest that the basal ganglia are some of the "chief brain error processors" that ensure adequate completion of information processing for cognitive control. A disruption in dopamine signal caused by alcohol in these brain regions disinhibits adequate processing of information (Nieuwenhuis et al., 2003; Ridderinkhof et al., 2003; Umhau et al., 2003; Holroyd & Yeung 2003; Holroyd & Coles 2002; Hester et al., 2005; Garavan et al., 2002; Easdon et al., 2005).

6. Mechanism & processes of alcohol's effect on the error monitoring and processing functions of the Basal Ganglia: The ARGD-EMPS hypothesis revisited and redefined

How does alcohol exert its action on the error monitoring and processing capacity of the basal ganglia? This is a question that is virtually left unanswered as the traditional theories of error processing do not provide suitable answers. Of all the theories of error monitoring and processing, only the hypothesis of alcohol-related glucose-dependent system of error monitoring & processing (ARGD-EMPS hypothesis) gives a somewhat precise definition of how alcohol affects the EMPS, although, even ARGD-EMPS hypothesis has its short-comings. For one reason, while ARGD-EMPS hypothesis proposes an indirect mechanism of alcohol's action on the EMPS, a direct pathway is also possible. Secondly, the hypothesis considers competency of glucose homeostasis regulation to affect the ACC primarily, and then, consequently, affecting other components of the system. Finally, the effect of alcohol on the EMPS might take a much longer time than expected.

The ARGD-EMPS hypothesis which explains the general processes and mechanisms of alcohol-related disruption of the EMPS, suggests that the disruption of EMPS by alcohol might be indirect and realized through its effect on the competency of glucose homeostasis regulation (Welcome et al., 2010) (also see Fig. 2). The major postulates of this hypothesis hold that the error processing capacity of the ACC depends on the blood-brain glucose proportionality level, which affects the dopaminergic system as a major component of the EMPS (Pizzagalli et al., 2003; Umhau et al., 2003; Goldstein et al., 2007).

From figure 2, one can notice that one of the central dogma of the ARGD-EMPS hypothesis is the degree of glucose homeostasis (allostasis is a better terminology) regulation in blood

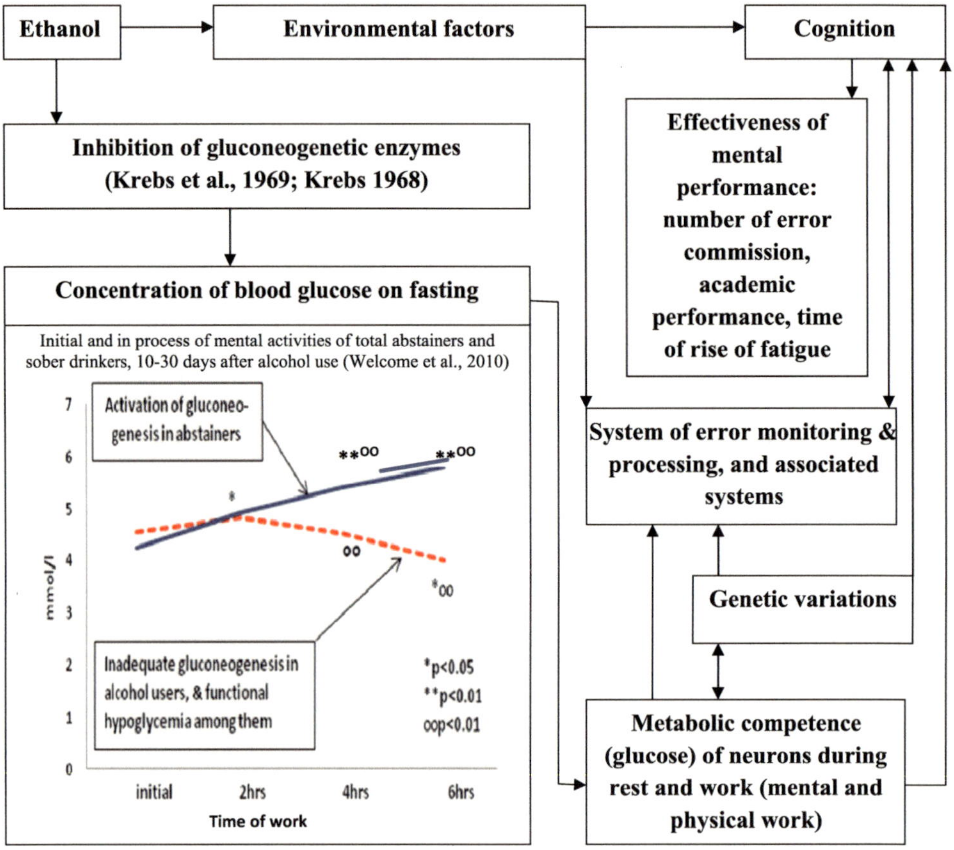

Significance level: *in relation to the initial level; °°in relation to the parameters of the opposite group.

References to figure: Welcome et al., 2010 & 2011; Krebs 1968; Nieuwenhuis et al., 2004; Ridderinkhof et al., 2002; Holroyd & Yeung 2003; Montague et al., 1996; Carter et al., 1998; Bello & Hajnal 2006; Haltia et al., 2007; Williams et al., 2007; de Galan et al., 2006; Calhoun et al., 2004; Umhau et al., 2003; Haight & Keatinge 1973; Krebs et al., 1969; Wick et al. 1998

Figure 2. Ethanol affects the functions of the EMPS by altering the brain and blood glucose levels through its action on the mechanisms (gluconeogentic etc) that regulate the blood-brain glucose concentration (the effect is also evident among sober individual, even for 10-30 days after alcohol use. Genetic variations in dopamine, GABA receptors can also affect the activities of the EMPS. The resultant effects of all these components on EMPS indirectly affect cognition, at the same time as the level of cognition can affect the activity level of EMPS. Ethanol as a component of environmental factors can affect cognition. Ethanol reduces the glycemic level of alcohol users, especially in tasks requiring high cognitive control, and subsequently affecting EMPS.

and brain. Disorder in glucose homeostasis regulation in blood, and in the brain, especially under long-term intensive mental activities in alcohol users is the basis for the formulation of the ARGD-EMPS hypothesis. Importantly, road traffic, and aviation catastrophes, glucose allostasis regulation might stand out to be a major reason. Unarguably, long-hour driving and airplane control requires significant cognitive control, judgment. In alcohol users (even after 7-30 days of alcohol use), this cognitive control might malfunction by increase in error commission, especially after long period (~4 hrs and above) of driving or control. The situation might be pronounced for young people. Besides, catastrophic cases of vehicle accidents involving alcohol use are more prevalent among young people, especially among students (Del Rio Carmen et al., 2001). While alcohol's time-dose effects are largely studied, data about the time-response effect in healthy young individuals remain scanty. In our recent work (Welcome et al., 2011), for the first time, we were able to identify statistically, a lowering of glycemic allostasis regulation in young sober healthy students who use alcohol episodically in moderate doses. This lowering in glycemia correlated significantly with cognitive functions. The study was conducted after one week to a month abstinence period for alcohol users to extensively study the time-response effect of alcohol.

6.1. Relationship between alcohol use and cognitive functions

In the study (Welcome et al., 2011; tables 1, 2, and 3), analysis of the parameters of effectiveness of active attention (a function of cognitive control) in the participants was conducted according the results of the test "Correction Probe" and was based on the number of error commission in the test. Number of error commission by the episodic alcohol users in the test "Correction Probe" was by 5.43 ($P<0.02$) – 12.77 ($P<0.005$) times higher compared to the non-alcohol users in all phases (tests) of the experiment (table 1). Number of error commission by alcohol episodic alcohol users significantly exceeded in all phases of mental activities (after 2, 4 and 6 hrs) and was after 6 hrs from the start +17.6±5.8 errors ($P<0.01$), or 218.4 % in relation to the initial number (table 1). Among the non-alcohol users, the number of errors did not change and remained low and stable during the experiment.

The number of errors in the test "Correction Probe" also allowed to analyze a very important property of active attention – concentration which is the possibility to focus on ongoing activities so as to minimize error commission to ≤ 5 errors in the test "Correction Probe". This property of attention was especially expressed among the non-alcohol users (in 87.5 – 100.0% cases), both in the initial (1st) test and in course (dynamics) of carrying out mental activities (table 1). Among alcohol users attention concentration or focus was retained only in 4 (>5 errors in the test "Correction Probe") out of 19 persons. As a result of this, the estimated relative probability of maintaining proper attention concentration or focus (≤ 5 errors in the test "Correction Probe") among non-alcohol users was 4.15 times ($P<0.002$; $\chi^2=10.296$) higher, than among their colleagues who use alcohol. According to the measure of carrying out mental activities, concentration of attention among the alcohol users decreased and remained low even after two hrs of rest. As a result, the risk of error commission of more than 5 in the test "Correction Probe" and lowering of the concentration of attention among the alcohol users increased from 6.29 to 8.00 ($P<0.001$; $\chi^2=17.459$) times compared to the non-alcohol users.

Test number and time of carrying out the test	Number of errors in the test "CP"		Dynamics of number of errors	
	group № 1	group № 2	group № 1	group № 2
1st, initial (M ± m),	**2.8 ± 0.8**	**15.2 ± 3.5 ۞**	---	---
P,t ۞ at df=7 – to the parameters of № 1		P<0.02; t=3.471		
2nd, after 2hrs of work (M±m)	**2.4 ± 0.7**	**18.2 ± 4.1 ۞**	**– 0,4 ± 0,5**	**+ 3.0 ± 1.4 ***
P, t * - to the initial value of its own group	P>0.05	P>0.05	P>0.05	P<0.05;t=2.143; df=18
P,t ۞ at df=7 – to the initial value of № 1		P<0.01; t=3.847		P>0.05; t=2.272
3rd, after 4hrs of work (M±m)	**3.1 ± 0.7**	**25.1 ± 4.9 ۞**	**+ 0.3 ± 0.8**	**+ 9.0 ± 3.5*۞**
P, t * - to the initial value of its own group	P>0.05	P>0.05	P>0.05	P<0.02;t=2.586; df=17
P,t ۞ at df=7 – to the value of № 1		P<0.005; t=4.477		P<0.05; t=2.415
4th, after 6hrs of work (M±m)	**2.6 ± 0.7**	**33.2 ± 7.1 *۞**	**– 0.2 ± 0.6**	**+17.6±5.8*۞**
P, t *- to the initial value of its own group	P>0.05	P<0.05;t=2.288; df=17	P>0.05	P<0.01;t=3.034; df=17
P,t ۞ at df=7 – to the value of № 1		P<0.005; t=4.315		P<0.02; t=3.052
5th, after 2 hrs of rest (M±m)	**2.5 ± 1.1**	23.3 ± 4.2 ۞	**– 0.3 ± 0.9**	+ 13.2 ± 6.9
P,t ۞ at df=7 – to the value of № 1		P<0.005; t=4.755		P>0.05

Note: group № 1 –non-alcohol users (8 persons); group № 2 – alcohol users (19 persons). Significance of differences was calculated with Student's t-test: * – significance of the differences in relation to the parameters of students in its own group on the first test (initial parameters in its own group); ۞– significance of the differences in relation to analogical parameters of non-alcohol users in the same phase (number) of testing.

Table 1. Number of errors and effectiveness of attention in the test "Correction Probe" (CP)

These facts strongly suggest that alcohol use, even episodic in moderate doses leads to long-term (1 – 4 weeks) negative effect on the state of cognitive functions in sober young people. This is manifested through decrease in the concentration of attention and worsening of the processes of active attention (table 1), processes of thinking, different types of memory resulting in inability to preserve proper level of mental performance for a long period of time and relative rise of fatigue. In addition, analysis of academic performance (which might represent a factor of cognitive functions) show decrease in the effectiveness to sit for examinations only among the alcohol users.

6.2. Episodic alcohol use, glycemia and cognitive functions: What are the possible connections?

Research data on the chief role of glucose in energy supply for neurons and the inhibition of gluconeogenesis during acute or chronic alcohol poisoning have been repeatedly reported (Krebs 1968; Krebs et al., 1969; Goodlett & Horn 2001). The result of our study suggests that that inhibition of gluconeogenesis by ethanol is a fairly long process (1 – 4 weeks, and may possibly last longer until complete recovery of gluconeogenetic enzymes by de novo synthesis).

Blood sampling	Concentration of glucose in capillary blood (M±m), mmol/l		
	All participants, n=27	Non-alcohol users, group № 1, n=8	Alcohol users, group № 2, n=19
Initial, before work	**4.45 ± 0.12**	**4.24 ± 0.19**	**4.54 ± 0.15**
⊛ t , St. to abstainers group №1	P > 0.05		P > 0.05
After 2hrs of work	**4.85±0.10 ***	**4.91±0.15 ***	**4.82±0.13**
* t , St. to the initial	P<0.02;t=2.548;df=26	P<0.05;t=2.792;df=7	P>0.05;t=1.914;df=18
⊛ t ,St. to № 1	P > 0.05		P > 0.05
Dynamics to initial	**+0.40±0.08 ***	**+0.67±0.08 ***	**+0.28±0.10*⊛**
* t , St. to the initial	P<0.001;t=5.000;df=26	P<0.001;t=8.375;df=7	P<0.02;t=2.800;df=18
⊛ t ,St. to № 1	P<0.05;t=2.385;df=7		P<0.02;t=3.042;df=7
After 4hrs of work	**4.79±0.12**⊛n=26	**5.40±0.18 ***	**4.52±0.11**⊛n=18
* t , St. to the initial	P>0.05;t=2.000;df=25	P<0.005;t=4.462;df=7	P>0.05;t=0.091;df=17
⊛ t ,St. to № 1	P<0.05;t=2.385;df=7		P<0.005;t=4.190;df=7
Dynamics to initial	**+0.35±0.15 *⊛**	**+1.16±0.17 ***	**–0.01±0.14**⊛n=18
* t , St. to the initial	P<0.05;t=2.333;df=25	P<0.001;t=6.824;df=7	P>0.05;t=0.007;df=17
⊛ t ,St. to № 1	P<0.01;t=3.568;df=7		P<0.002;t=5.294;df=7
After 6hrs of work	**4.54±0.21**⊛n=26	**5.78±0.13 ***	**3.99±0.18**⊛n=18
* t , St. to initial	P>0.05;t=0.372;df=25	P<0.001;t=6.696;df=7	P<0.05;t=2.347;df=17
⊛ t ,St. to № 1	P<0.005;t=5.020;df=7		P<0.001;t=8.063;df=7
Dynamics to initial	**+0.10±0.25 ⊛**	**+1.54±0.16 ***	**–0.55±0.24 ***⊛n=18
* t , St. to the initial	P>0.05;t=0.400;df=25	P<0.001;t=9.625;df=7	P<0.05;t=2.292;df=17
⊛ t ,St. to № 1	P<0.005;t=4.848;df=7		P<0.001;t=7.232;df=7

Note: * – differences are significant in relation to the initial level of glycemia in its own group before work (the first blood sampling) with respect to Student's t criterion (St.). ⊛ – differences are significant in relation to the level of glycemia among the non-alcohol users on the same phase of blood sampling. n – number of participants in the group.

Table 2. Initial parameters and dynamics of blood glucose in capillary blood of all respondents in a condition of long-term, intensive mental activities

Inadequate level of glycemia for long-term energy supply for actively working neurons, which is accompanied by lowering of their activities and subsequently a decline in cognitive function, even in sober respondents could be due to inadequacy in the activity of gluconeogenetic enzymes. The observed disorders in glucose metabolism may be expressed in conditions of intense functional workloads, for example, mental activities, imposed on sober respondents on fasting in the catabolic phase of metabolism. This assumption is confirmed by the result of studying the dynamics of glucose in the blood of hungry people with different attitudes to alcohol in a condition of long-term functional workload (on fasting) in the form of intensive 6 hrs mental activities (table 2).

The results of this study showed increase in the level of blood glucose in all 27 participants in the first 2 hrs of mental activities (figure 2; table 2) by +0.40 mmol/l (P<0.001): among the non-alcohol users – +0.67 mmol/l (P<0.001), in the sober respondents – +0.28 mmol/l (P<0.02). Further dynamics of glycemic level in the remaining 26 participants (one participant declined from continuing the experiment as a result of fatigue after 3hrs from the start), that continued the experiment was different from that in the first two hours of work.

Increase in the level of glycemia after 4 hrs of mental work was +0.35 mmol/l ($P<0.05$) compared to the initial level; by 0.05 mmol/l less compared to the level after 2hrs (table 2). After 6hrs of mental work average glycemic level increased slightly, but was not different from the level at the first blood sampling, although was less compared to the level after 2 and 4hrs of work (table 2). This suggests that the process of using glucose is more pronounced than the process of its formation (after 4hrs of work) and entrance of glucose into blood: the exhaustion of reserves and stimulation of gluconeogenesis for the maintenance of proper level of blood glucose, to providing the energy requirements of actively working cells and organs. Cessation of increase of glycemic level after 4hrs of work among the majority of respondents and its normalization after 6hrs of mental activities was because of the differences in the dynamics of this important parameter in all participants (figure 2; table 2).

In all non-alcohol users, in all phases of the experiment, there was increase in the glycemic level. The average increase of the glycemic level in relation to the initial level was +0.67 mmol/l ($P<0.05$) after 2 hrs, +1.16 mmol/l ($P<0.001$) after 4hrs, and +1.54 mmol/l ($P<0.001$) after 6hrs. Positive dynamics of increase in the glycemic level among the non-alcohol users in a condition of active use of glucose by the brain imply a high reserve of gluconeogenesis amongst them and its intense stimulation in a condition of long-term mental activities. If one should bring into mind the fact that [in condition of catabolism, gluconeogenesis determines the quantity of glucose that enters the blood (De Galan et al., 2006; Krebs 1968), and that glucose use by the brain during mental activities increases at least by 12% (Madsen et al., 1995; Di Nuzzo et al., 2009), that increase in glycemic level after 6hrs of work among the non-alcohol users was 36.3% /table 2/], then calculation of shows increase in the activity of gluconeogenesis by approximately 1.53 times in relation to the initial level.

Amongst the group 2 students, dynamics of glycemia after 4 and 6 hrs of mental activities were significantly different from that of the non-alcohol users (table 2). So, increase in blood glucose in the sober respondents after 2 hrs of mental work (+0.28 mmol/l /$P<0.02$/) was replaced by a decrease after 4 hrs of mental work and the development of hypoglycemia (3.99 mmol/l /$P<0.05$/) for capillary blood (table 2) after 6hrs of mental activities. Three students had neuroglycopenia at the end of the experiment, because their blood glucose level was less than 3.0 mmol/l. This is a confirmation that the reserve of gluconeogenesis in sober individuals is significantly decreased compared to the non-alcohol users.

Pearson linear correlation analysis showed the presence of significant (linear, positive) linkages between the glycemic level and effectiveness of cognitive function in all tests after 4 and 6 hrs of mental activities (table 3). In addition, after 4 and 6 hrs of work, there was a significant negative correlation between blood glucose and number of error commission in the test "Correction Probe" (table 3). Calculation of the coefficient of determination (r^2) shows that the proportion by contribution of glycemic level and effectiveness of cognitive functions in all tests were 11.8% ($P<0.05$) after 4hrs and 15.6% ($P<0.05$) after 6hrs of work. The calculated percentage of the effect of blood glucose on the parameters of mental performance clearly does not agree with literature data (Madsen et al., 1995; Di Nuzzo et al., 2009) on the positive effect of glycemia as energy source for neurons (on the average ~ 35%). One can assume that the effect of glycemic control on cognitive functions carry a linear character, not a curvilinear one, especially if we consider the fact that indirect source of glucose to the majority of neurons is through glial cells.

6.3. Effect of glycemic control on error commission

The conducted calculation of the coefficient of correlational relationship of Pearson "η" for the analysis of the degree of curvilinear linkage showed the presence of one-sided effect (with average strength) of glycemia on effectiveness of cognitive function and number of error commission in the test "Correction Probe" for the analysis of mental performance and fatigue in the participants (table 3). Calculations of the coefficient of determination η^2, or r^2 confirms with sufficient evidence of a direct role of glycemic level (26.0% on fasting at rest; 30.0 – 36.7% on fasting during mental work) amongst all factors, contributing to mental performance and the state of cognitive functions. The proportion by contribution of glycemia (26.0 – 36.7 % /P<0.01/) in the provision of brain functions (mental performance of a person) closely agree with the value (35.0 %) (Madsen et al., 1995; Di Nuzzo et al., 2009) for the provision of energy for neurons in different conditions. Therefore, sufficient concentration of blood glucose is one of the major factors of high mental performance and high state of cognitive processes.

Type of correlation, pair of correlating parameters	Values of correlation coefficients			
	Before work	During work		
	Initial (1st)	After 2hrs (2nd)	After 4hrs (3rd)	After 6hrs (4th)
Participants	n=27	n=27	n=26	n=26
$r_{Pearson}$Gl– NO in the test "CP", ⊙	$r = -0.01$ $P = 0.994$	$r = -0.165$ $P = 0.206$	$r = -0.364$ ⊙ $P = 0.034$	$r = -0.398$ ⊙ $P = 0.022$
$\eta_{Pearson}$ Gl – NO in the test "CP", ▪ Effect of Gl on NO	$\eta = 0.510$ ▪ $P < 0.01$ $\eta^2 \cdot 100\% = 26.0\%$▪	$\eta = 0.548$ ▪ $P < 0.001$ $\eta^2 \cdot 100\% = 30.0\%$▪	$\eta = 0.606$ ▪ $P < 0.001$ $\eta^2 \cdot 100\% = 36.7\%$▪	$\eta = 0.556$ ▪ $P < 0.001$ $\eta^2 \cdot 100\% = 30.9\%$▪

Note: Gl – glucose (concentration of glucose in capillary blood); NO – number of errors; test "CP" – test "Correction Probe"; r – linear correlation coefficient of Pearson; η – curvilinear correlation coefficient of Pearson; ⊙– significance of linkage between the parameters with respect to "r" linear correlation coefficient of Pearson set at P≤0,05; ▪ – significance of one-sided effect of glucose on number of error committed by the participants on the test "CP", in relation to "η" curvilinear correlation coefficient of Pearson set at P≤0,05. Proportion of interrelationship of the analyzed parameters were calculated based on the coefficient of determination (r^2) [see Welcome et al., 2011]. Tests were conducted together with the blood sampling of glucose in each phase of the experiment.

Table 3. Effect of glycemia on the parameters of cognitive functions and the functional state of the participants

The hypoglycemic effect of acute alcohol administration has been known for decades. As reported by Hans Krebs and associates, alcohol reduces the activeness of gluconeogenetic enzymes (Krebs 1968; Krebs et al., 1969). We had reported that the negative effect of chronic (episodic) alcohol use on gluconeogenesis maybe long-term (might last even for 10-30 days after alcohol use), and might be noticed under long-term mental work (4-6 hrs), especially in task requiring high cognitive control (Welcome et al., 2011; Fig. 2).

The fact that decrease in neuronal gluconeogenesis (leading to ↓blood-brain glucose level) caused by alcohol consumption in a cognitive task might affect the activities of the EMPS by increase in the number of error commission is evident in the hypothalamic control of blood and brain glucose levels (Welcome et al., 2010; Volkow et al., 2006). The blood glucose level increases with increase in dopamine level on fasting (Umhau et al., 2003). Effect of glucose on dopamine is realized through the activities of GLUT- 2 receptor located in hypothalamic neurons (Umhau et al., 2003; Williams et al., 2007; Pizzagalli 2003).

The basal ganglia and hypothalamus are actively engaged with the brain regions of cognitive control to adequately carryout a task to meet set aims. To meet the set aims, one of the control mechanisms is to avoid error commission. However, in rare circumstances error commission can be an adaptive mechanism for safety, and accommodation, and may result from neuronal selectivity pattern (Gehring et al., 1993; Hester et al., 2005; Bello & Hajnal 2006). The increased error commission associated with alcohol consumption is related to decrease in dopaminergic functions (Nieuwenhuis et al., 2002; Holroyd & Yeung 2003), which is caused by decreased competence of glucose allostasis regulation (Welcome et al., 2010, 2011).

It is possible to assume that functional hypoglycemia among sober individuals (within a period of 30 days after alcohol use) in a condition of mental activities may lead to disorders in dopamine metabolism and subsequently cause disruption of EMPS through increase in erroneous actions.

According to the ARGD-EMPS hypothesis, the disruption of the EMPS is related to the competency of glucose allostasis regulation, which in turn may determine the dopamine level as a major component of the EMPS (Welcome et al., 2010).

Blood and brain glucose levels play a vital role in error commission, and are related to error commission, monitoring and processing through the modulation of the activity of the dopaminergic system (Volkow et al., 2006; Umhau et al., 2003; Williams et al., 2007; Pizzagalli 2003). In fact, decreased glucose metabolism in ACC closely correlates with the results of neurophysiological tests (Pizzagalli et al., 2003).

The ARGD-EMPS hypothesis was put forward based on recent evidences, which suggest that alcohol's action on error monitoring ad processing is related to its action on glucose homeostasis regulation, especially in tasks requiring high cognitive control (Welcome et al., 2010). In addition, the number of errors committed in an experiment is inversely correlated with the glycemic levels, especially among alcohol users (Welcome et al., 2010, 2011; Fig. 2). In addition, correlation analysis between academic performance and the number of errors committed by alcohol users in high-level cognitive task is also a confirmation (Welcome et al., 2010, 2011; Fig. 2).

7. Conclusion

The basal ganglia represent a crucial relay station for error monitoring and processing between several brain regions including emotional and cognitive brain areas. The disruption of error monitoring and processing by alcohol might not follow an indirect pathway only, but also a direct one. Indirect effect of alcohol may be possible through the processing capacity of the basal ganglia by affecting other brain areas connected to the basal ganglia; action of alcohol metabolites (acetaldehyde; acetate; protein-, lipid-, enzyme-, and DNA-adducts of alcohol) on the processing of information in the basal ganglia and/or associated brain pathways; and its action on neuromediators that modulate the processing of information in the basal ganglia and/or associated brain pathways. The direct effect might be attained if alcohol reach the basal ganglia and causes disruption of cellular processes including information processing. The effect is a change in effectiveness of cognitive functions, error commission in the macro world. The effect of alcohol on the basal ganglia's error monitoring and processing capacity might last for several days after alcohol use (up to 30 days). This effect might be noted, especially under long-term intensive mental activities requiring high cognitive control, when the glucose reserves in the body cannot support long-term actively working neurons, and this may lead to disorders in dopamine metabolism and subsequently cause disruption of EMPS through decrease in effectiveness of cognitive functions, increase in erroneous actions.

8. Future research

Future research will examine both the electrophysiological (ECG, ERN etc.) and radiological (PET, etc) parameters of dose-time response effect of alcohol in details. In the initial stage, animal models will be used to research the basis and to test how alcohol affect specific neuron or group of neurons in basal ganglia-thalamo-cortico-limbic pathways. Other pathways with indirect connections to the basal ganglia whose dysfunctions may necessary lead to a decrease in basal ganglia function will also be examined. A knockout of the alcohol pocket-receptor might also reveal useful information about the indirect effect of alcohol on error monitoring and processing.

Author details

M.O. Welcome and V.A. Pereverzev
Belarusian State Medical University, Minsk, Belarus

9. References

Aarts K, Pourtois G. Anxiety not only increases, but also alters early error-monitoring functions. *Cogn Affect Behav Neurosci*. 2010;10 (4): 479-492.

Amodio DM, Kubota JT, Harmon-Jones E, Devine PG. Alternative mechanisms for regulating racial responses according to internal vs external cues. *SCAN*. 2006; 1: 26–36.

Aparicio P, Diedrichsen J, Ivry RB. Effects of focal basal ganglia lesions on timing and force control. *Brain Cognition*. 2005; 58: 62–74.

Bello NT, Hajnal A. Alterations in blood glucose levels under hyperinsulinemia affect accumbens dopamine. *Physiol Behav* 2006; 88: 138–145.

Berry EL, Nicolson RI, Foster JK, Behrmann M, Sagar HJ. Slowing of Reaction Time in Parkinson's Disease: The Involvement of the Frontal Lobes. *Neuropsychologia*. 1999; 37: 676-684.

Beste C, Saft C, Andrich J, Gold R, Falkenstein M. Error Processing in Huntington's Disease. *PLoS ONE*. 2006; 1(1): e86.

Beste C, Saft C, Andrich J, Gold R, Falkenstein M. Stimulus-Response Compatibility in Huntington's Disease: A Cognitive-Neurophysiological Analysis. *J Neurophysiol*. 2008; 99:1213-1223.

Beste C, Saft C, Andrich J, Mu¨ ller T, Gold R, Falkenstein M. Time Processing in Huntington's Disease: A Group-Control Study. *PLoS ONE*. 2007; 2 (12):e1263.

Beste C, Willemsen R, Saft C, Falkenstein M. Error processing in normal aging and in basal ganglia disorders. *Neuroscience*. 2009; 159: 143–149.

Bocquillon P, Bourriez J-L, Palmero-Soler E, Deste´e A, Defebvre L, Derambure P, Dujardin K. Role of Basal Ganglia Circuits in Resisting Interference by Distracters: A swLORETA Study. *PLoS ONE*. 2012; 7 (3): e34239.

Botvinick MM, Braver TS, Barch DM, Carter CS, Cohen JD. Conflict monitoring and cognitive control. *Psychol Rev*. 2001; 108 (3): 624-652.

Botvinick MM, Cohen JD, Carter CS. Conflict monitoring and anterior cingulate cortex: an update. *Trends Cogn Sci*. 2004; 8 (12): 539-546.

Buhler R, Pestalozzi D, Hess M, von Wartburg J.-P. Immunohistochemical Localization of Alcohol Dehydrogenase in Human Kidney, Endocrine Organs and Brain. *Pharmacol Biochem Behav*. 1983; 18 (1): 55-59.

Calhoun VD, Pekar JJ, Pearlson GD. Alcohol intoxication effects on simulated driving: exploring alcohol-dose effects on brain activation using functional MRI. *Neuropsychopharmacology* 2004; 29: 2097-2107.

Carter CS, Braver TS, Barch DM, Botvinick MM, Noll D, Cohen JD. Anterior cingulate cortex, error detection, and the online monitoring of performance. *Science* 1998; 280: 747-749.

Charlesworth JD, Warren TL, Brainard MS. Covert skill learning in a cortical-basal ganglia circuit. *Nature*. 2012; 486: 251–255.

De Galan BE, Schouwenberg BJ, Tack CJ, Smits P. Pathophysiology and management of recurrent hypoglycaemia and hypoglycaemia unawareness in diabetes. *Neth J Med* 2006; 64: 269-279.

Deitrich, Zimatkin S, Pronko S. Oxidation of Ethanol in the Brain and Its Consequences. *Alcohol Res Health*. 2006; 29 (4): 266-273.

Del Rio Carmen M, Gonzalez-Luque JC, Alvarez FJ. *Alcohol Alcohol*. 2001; 36 (3): 256-261.

Dhar M, Wiersema JR, Pourtois G. Cascade of Neural Events Leading from Error Commission to Subsequent Awareness Revealed Using EEG Source Imaging. *PLoS ONE*. 2011; 6 (5): e19578.

Di Nuzzo M, Giove F, Bruno Maraviglia. A biochemical framework for modeling the functional metabolism of the human brain. Biophys BioEngin Letters 2009; 2 (2): 1-26.

Easdon C, Izenberg A, Armilio ML, Yu H, Alain C. Alcohol consumption impairs stimulus- and error-related processing during a Go/No-Go Task. *Brain Res Cogn Brain Res*. 2005; 25: 873–883.

Endrass T, Klawohn J, Preuss J, Kathmann N. Temporospatial dissociation of Pesubcomponentsforperceivedandunperceivederrors. *Front Hum Neurosci*. 2012; 6 (Article178): 1-10.

Falkenstein M, Hohnsbein J, Hoormann J. Event-related potential correlates of errors in reaction tasks. In: G Karmos, M Molnar, V Csepe, I Czigler, JE Desmedt, eds. *Perspectives of Event-related Potentials Research*. Amsterdam: Elsevier. 1995; 287–296.

Falkenstein M, Hoormann J, Christ S, Hohnsbein J. ERP components on reaction errors and their functional significance: a tutorial. *Biol Psychol*. 2000; 51 (2-3): 87-107.

Fein G, Chang M. Smaller feedback ERN amplitudes during the BART are associated with a greater family history density of alcohol problems in treatment-naïve alcoholics. *Drug Alcohol Depend*. 2008; 92 (1-3): 141-148.

Franken IHA, van Strien JW, Kuijpers I. Evidence for a deficit in the salience attribution to errors in smokers. *Drug Alcohol Depend*. 2010; 106 (2-3): 181-185.

Garavan H, Ross TJ, Murphy K, Roche RA, Stein EA. Dissociable executive functions in the dynamic control of behavior: inhibition, error detection, and correction. *NeuroImage*. 2002; 17: 1820–1829.

Garavan H, Ross TJ, Murphy K, Roche RA, Stein EA. Dissociable executive functions in the dynamic control of behavior: inhibition, error detection, and correction. *Neuroimage*. 2002;17 (4):1820-1829.

Gehring WJ, Fencsik DE. Functions of the medial frontal cortex in the processing of conflict and errors. *J Neurosci*. 2001; 21: 9430–9437.

Gehring WJ, Goss B, Coles M, Meyer D, Donchin E. A neural system for error detection and compensation. *Psychol Sci*. 1993; 4: 385–390.

Giesbrecht T, Geraerts E, Merckelbach H. Dissociation, memory commission errors, and heightened autonomic reactivity. *Psychiatr Res*. 2007; 150: 277–285.

Goldstein RZ, Tomasi D, Rajaram S, et al. Role of anterior cingulate and medial orbitofrontal cortex in processing drug cues in cocaine addiction. *Neuroscience*. 2007; 144: 1153– 1159.

Goodlett CR, Horn KH. Mechanism of Alcohol Induced Damage to the Developing Nervous System. Alcohol Res Health 2001; 25 (3): 175-184.

Haight JS, Keatinge WR. Failure of thermoregulation in the cold during hypoglycaemia induced by exercise and ethanol. *J Physiol* 1973; 229: 87-97.

Haltia LT, Rinne JO, Merisaari H, Maguire RP, Savontaus E, Helin S, Någren K, et al. Effects of intravenous glucose on dopaminergic function in the human brain in vivo. *Synapse* 2007; 61: 748 – 756.

Hester R, Foxe JJ, Molholm S, Shpaner M, Garavan H. Neural mechanisms involved in error processing: a comparison of errors made with and without awareness. *NeuroImage*. 2005; 27: 602–608.

Holroyd CB, Coles MGH. The neural basis of human error processing: reinforcement learning, dopamine, and the error-related negativity. *Psychol Rev*. 2002; 109: 679–709.

Holroyd CB, Praamstra P, Plat E, Coles MGH. Spared error-related potentials in mild to moderate Parkinson's disease. *Neuropsychologia*. 2002; 1419: 1-9.

Holroyd CB, Praamstra P, Plat E, Coles MGH. Spared error-related potentials in mild to moderate Parkinson's disease. *Neuropsychologia*. 2002; 40: 2116–2124.

Holroyd CB, Yeung N. Alcohol and error processing. *Trends Neurosci* 2003; 26: 402- 404.

Hurst JW. Cognitive Errors (Can They Be Prevented?). *Am J Cardiol*. 2008; 101 (10): 1513-1517.

Jin DZ, Fujii N, Graybiel AM. Neural representation of time in cortico-basal ganglia circuits. *PNAS*. 2009; 106 (45): 19156–19161.

Krebs HA. The effects of ethanol on the metabolic activities of the liver. *Adv Enzyme Regul* 1968; 6: 467-480.

Krebs, HA, Freedland RA, Hems R, Stubbs M. Inhibition of hepatic gluconeogenesis by ethanol. *Biochem J* 1969; 112:117-124.

Krigolson OE, Holroyd CB. Hierarchical error processing: different errors, different systems. *Brain Res*. 2007; 1155: 70-80.

Madsen PL, Hasselbalch SG, Hageman LP, Olsen KS, Bulow J, Holm S, Wildschioedtz G, Paulson OB, Lassen NA. Persistent resetting of the cerebral oxygen/glucose uptake ratio by brain activation: evidence obtained with the KetySchmidt technique. *J Cereb Blood Flow Metabol* 1995; 15: 485-491.

Marco-Pallarés J, Camara E, Münte TF, Rodríguez-Fornells A. Neural mechanisms underlying adaptive actions after slips. *J Cogn Neurosci*. 2008; 20 (9): 1595-610.

Mathalon DH, Whitfield SL, Ford JM. Anatomy of an error: ERP and fMRI, *Biol Psychol*. 2003; 64: 119–141.

Mitler MM, Carskadon MA, Czeisler CA, Dement WC, Dinges DF, Graeber RC. Catastrophes, Sleep, and Public Policy: Consensus Report. *Sleep*. 1988; 11(1): 100–109.

Montague PR, Dayan P, Sejnowsk TJ. A framework for mesencephalic dopamine systems based on predictive Hebbian learning. *J Neurosci* 1996; 76: 1936-1947.

Münte TF, Heldmann M, Hinrichs H, et al. Nucleus accumbens is involved in human action monitoring: evidence from invasive electrophysiological recordings. *Hum Neurosci*. 2008; 1 (11): 1-6.

Nick Y, Botvinick MM, Cohen JD. The neural basis of error detection: Conflict monitoring and the error-related negativity. *Psychol Rev*. 2004; 111 (4): 931-959.

Nieuwenhuis S, Holroyd CB, Mol N, Coles MG. Reinforcement related brain potentials from medial frontal cortex: origins and functional significance. *Neurosci Biobehav Rev* 2004; 28: 441-448.

Nieuwenhuis S, Ridderinkhof KR, Talsma D, et al. A computational account of altered error processing in older age: dopamine and the error-related negativity. *Cogn Affect Behav Neurosci*. 2002; 2: 19–36.

Nieuwenhuis S, Yeung N, van den Wildenberg W, Ridderinkhof KR. Electrophysiological correlates of anterior cingulate function in a Go/NoGo task: Effects of response conflict and trial-type frequency. *Cogn Affect Behav Neurosci.* 2003; 3: 17-26.

Olvet DM, Hajcak G. The error-related negativity (ERN) and psychopathology: Toward an endophenotype. *Clin Psychol Rev.* 2008: 28 (8): 1343-1354.

Pailing PE, Segalowitz SJ. The error-related negativity as a state and trait measure: Motivation, personality, and ERPs in response to errors. *Psychophysiology.* 2004; 41(1): 84-84.

Pizzagalli DA, Oakes TR, Davidson RJ. Coupling of theta activity and glucose metabolism in the human rostral anterior cingulate cortex: an EEG/PET study of normal and depressed subjects. Psychophysiology. 2003; 40: 939 –949.

Pontifex MB, Scudder MR, Brown ML, O'Leary KC, Wu C-T, Themanson JR, Hillman CH. On the number of trials necessary for stabilization of error-related brain activity across the life span. *Psychophysiology.* 2010; 47: 767–773.

Quertemont E. Genetic polymorphism in ethanol metabolism: acetaldehyde contribution to alcohol abuse and alcoholism. *Mol Psychiatry.* 2004; 9: 570–581.

Ridderinkhof KR, de Vlugt Y, Bramlage A, Spaan M, Elton M, Snel J, Band GP. Alcohol consumption impairs detection of performance errors in mediofrontal cortex. *Science* 2002; 298: 2209–2211.

Ridderinkhof KR, Nieuwenhuis S, Bashore TR. Errors are foreshadowed in brain potentials associated with action monitoring in cingulate cortex. *Neurosci Lett.* 2003; 348: 1-4.

S Gauggel, M Rieger, T-A Feghoff. Inhibition of ongoing responses in patients with Parkinson's disease. *J Neurol Neurosurg Psychiatry.* 2004; 75: 539–544.

Salvador M-A, Alfredo S-M. Cellular and Mitochondrial Effects of Alcohol Consumption. *Int J Environ Res Pub Health.* 2010; 7: 4281-4304.

Stevens MC, Kiehl KA, Pearlson GD, Calhoun VD. Brain Network Dynamics During Error Commission. *Hum Brain Mapp.* 2009; 30 (1): 24–37.

Suri R, Schultz W. A neural network with dopamine-like reinforcement signal that learns a spatial delayed response task. *Neuroscience.* 1999; 91: 871–890.

Umhau JC, Petrulis SG, Diaz R, Rawlings R, George DT. Blood glucose is correlated with cerebrospinal fluid neurotransmitter metabolites. *Neuroendocrinology* 2003; 78: 339– 343.

van Veen V, Carter CS. Error detection, correction, and prevention in the brain: a brief review of data and theories. *Clin EEG Neurosci.* 2006; 37 (4): 330-335.

Vocat R, Pourtois G, Vuilleumier P. Unavoidable errors: a spatio-temporal analysis of time-course and neural sources of evoked potentials associated with error processing in a speeded task. *Neuropsychologia.* 2008; 46 (10): 2545-55.

Volkow ND, Wang G-J, Franceschi D, et al. Low doses of alcohol substantially decrease glucose metabolism in the human brain. *NeuroImage.* 2006; 29: 295 – 301.

Welcome MO, Pereverzeva EV, Pereverzev VA. Long-term disorders of cognitive functions in sober people who episodically use alcohol, role of functional hypoglycemia and insufficiency of gluconeogenesis. *Bull Smolensk Med Acad* 2011; № 3: 2-20.

Welcome MO, Razvodovsky YE, Pereverzeva EV, Pereverzev VA. The effect of blood glucose concentration on the error monitoring and processing system in alcohol users during intensive mental activities. *Port Harcourt Med J*. 2011; 5 (3) 293-306.

Welcome MO, Razvodovsky YE, Pereverzeva EV, Pereverzev VA. The error monitoring and processing system in alcohol use. *IJCRIMPH*. 2010; 2 (10): 318-336.

Wick MJ, Mihic SJ, Ueno S, Mascia MP, Trudell JR, Brozowski SJ, Ye Q, Harrison NL, Harris RA. Mutations of g-aminobutyric acid and glycine receptors change alcohol cutoff: Evidence for an alcohol receptor? *Proc Natl Acad Sci USA*. 1998; 95: 6504–6509.

Williams JM, Owens WA, Turner GH, Saunders C, Dipace C, Blakely RD, France CP, et al. Hypoinsulinemia regulates amphetamine-induced reverse transport of dopamine. *PLoS Biol*. 2007; 5: e274.

Schulte T, Müller-Oehring EM, Strasburger H, Warzel H, Sabel BA. Acute effects of alcohol on divided and covert attention in men. *Psychopharmacology*. 2001; 154 (1): 61–69.

Ochoa G. Error Thresholds in Genetic Algorithms. *J Evolut Comput*. 2006; 14 (2): 157 – 182.

Takeuchi N, Poorthuis PH, Hogeweg P. Phenotypic error threshold; additivity and epistasis in RNA evolution. *BMC Evolut Biol*. 2005; 5:9. doi:10.1186/1471-2148-5-9.

Cohen SM, Ellwein LB. Genetic Errors, Cell Proliferation, and Carcinogenesis. *Cancer Res*. 1991; 51: 6493-6505.

Chapter 4

The Integrative Role of the Basal Ganglia

Clemens C.C. Bauer, Erick H. Pasaye,
Juan I. Romero-Romo and Fernando A. Barrios

Additional information is available at the end of the chapter

http://dx.doi.org/10.5772/54189

1. Introduction

Emergent experimental and clinical evidence supports the notion that the cortico-basal ganglia–thalamo-cortical loops progress along parallel circuits connecting cortical and subcortical regions subserving the processing of sensorimotor information, associative and affective knowledge [1]. In particular the role of the basal ganglia has long been known to be involved in motor control because of the marked deficits associated with their damage. However, the exact aspects of motor control that they have under normal conditions have not been clear at all. The traditional view is that the basal ganglia are involved in the selection and inhibition of action commands [2], but an increasing number of brain-imaging studies show that the basal ganglia, besides being involved in motor tasks are also involved in more integrative and cognitive processes such as mental imagery [3,4], sensory processing [5,6], planning [7], attention [8,9], and language [6,10,11]. This evidence supports the view that the basal ganglia output not only targets the primary sensory-motor cortices, but also specific areas of premotor and prefrontal cortex, which include the oculomotor area of the cortex, the dorsolateral prefrontal cortex, lateral orbitofrontal cortex, and anterior cingulate/medial orbitofrontal cortices [12]. Thus, having the ability to influence not only sensory-motor control, but also several different types of cognitive and limbic affective functions [12] which underlie complex and integrative processes such as self-awareness, introspective perspective of one's own self and consciousness [13]. This integrative role between lower afferent input and higher integrative and executive stages of information processing require an intact and closed loop of information flow to generate the primary experience of self and thus self-agency. Self-agency has tentatively been defined as the feeling of being the author of one's own actions [14]. Thus, when we move our arm, we know (a) that it is our arm and (b) that it is us, who moves the arm. One approach to understand the complex integration of afferent and efferent information processing and the integration in the self is the internal model theory of motor control [15]. According to this theory there are two functionally different components in the motor system, inverse and forward circuits. It is assumed that inverse models provide the motor commands necessary to achieve a desired consequence of an action, specified by higher-level goals (e.g., intentions). One is fully aware of the desired consequences of an action, but unaware of the motor programs per se. Forward models predict the sensory consequences of each motor program to be executed, an idea known as the efference copy, a model first put forward in von Holst and Mittelstaedt [16] and which has been extended in recent years with the "null" hypothesis of Ramachandran [17]. Accordingly, it is claimed that, whenever a motor program is issued, an efference copy is produced in parallel, this is, a prediction of the sensory consequences expected after the execution of the program based on exactly this efference copy. The internal model theory of motor control has been successfully applied to explain a whole variety of disorders related to the awareness of actions [for a review see 17] but the role played by the basal ganglia in this model has not been very clear. Here we follow this model extending it to the performance of a complex cognitive task, such as mental imaginary movement of a limb and the coexistent conscious awareness of just imagining it and actually refraining from moving it which involves exactly this subtle combination between the forward model requiring intact peripheral efferent/afferent information pathways and the inverse model requiring intact higher-level cortical areas which include the basal ganglia-thalamus-cortex pathway [19]. Moreover, we contrast the normal integrity of this forward/inverse model loop in healthy subjects with an abnormal open loop in amputees where an essential part of the loop has been disrupted. We thus argue that because of this abnormal and open loop involving the basal ganglia and the thalamocortical system the conscious awareness of the phantom phenomenon is created.

2. Problem statement

Waking up from anesthesia, an amputee faces the conflict in the experience of self, between the conscious vividness of his phantom limb (PL) and the lack of correlation with reality [20–23]. In the urge to discover whether he was actually amputated, the patient looks under the sheet for visual self-recognition and is, in a flash, confronted with this new reality of an absent limb. The resulting cognitive conflict between the seen embodiment and the felt one, in most cases carries on resulting in the perception of a ghost of their amputated limb as a phantom [24]. Giummarra et al. [20] report phantom limb experiences that include phenomena of (a) perception of bodily aspects of phantom limbs such as size (in relation to the intact limb), shape, posture, and telescoping (or shortening) of the phantom; (b) exteroceptive and proprioceptive sensations and (c) prosthesis embodiment. Early studies of phantom limb movement were carried out using combined techniques of EEG, MEG, and fMRI in order to locate its representation in the sensory-motor cortex [25–28] and in the cerebellum [29,30]. Later studies described the distinct functional anatomy of the mental representation of imaginary movements [31], during planning, visualizing, and motor intention [32], both in healthy subjects as well as in patients with different neural diseases. Other studies have centered on the difference between imaginary movement and executed movement [3,33]. A recent study by Diers et al. [34] showed activation in the supplementary motor area (SMA) cortex after PL imagined movement. And in a more recent study Pasaye et al. [35] have described nuerocorrelates of the PL perception using fMRI. Since the first conceptualization of the phenomenon of phantom limb in amputees in 1915, as the manifestation of the persistence of the body schema of the missing limb [36], many theories have arisen. Most of these theories suggest a central role of reorganization of the somatosensory cortex, others advocate for a perceptual completion [37], or the product of conflicting cues from central reorganizational changes [38]. Although some degree of sensory or motor impairment is constant, recent models of motor awareness suggest that the reduction in afferent information may be less critical than higher-level reorganization related to the subjective correlates of action planning and motor intention [15,39]. In contras, a number of studies of patients with amputated limbs encourage that a conscious perception of a body part by tactile stimulation does not necessarily require the integrity or even existence of the tactile receptors on the skin, or the body parts themselves. That is, the neural representation of the body in the brain is sufficient to elicit an awareness of the body part or tactile stimuli in the absence of its physical counterpart (e.g., the limbs themselves) [40]. We believe that the reduction or absence in afferent information is a key factor that in combination with higher-level reorganization generates the conscious awareness of the phantom phenomenon. Here we hypothesize that for the performance of a complex cognitive task, such as imaginary movement of a limb, and the concomitant conscious awareness of just imagining it and actually refraining from moving it, an involvement of a subtle combination between intact peripheric (efferent/afferent) information pathways and intact higher-level cortical areas (basal-ganglia-thalamus-cortex pathway) are needed [19]. In amputees, this normal combination of lower- and higher-level processes is disrupted and could be the underlying cause of conscious awareness of the phantom limb. This arrangement of processes was reported by Staub et al. [41], who found an increased blood oxygen level dependent (BOLD) signal in the Basal Ganglia-Thalamic-Motor-Cortex loop pathway during imaginary movement of a patient with chronic supernumerary phantom limb, which developed only in association with motor intent directed at a hemiplegic-anesthetic upper limb. Staub's finding is analogical to what Ramachandran proposes as the "null" signal hypothesis in the mirror neuron system (MNS), which prevents activity in the MNS from reaching the threshold for conscious awareness [17] or related to what Fitzgibbon et al. [42] suggests as the underlying cause in synesthesia for pain. We think that the logic behind Ramachandran's hypothesis is plausible, and if applied to an intact afferent somatosensory-proprioceptive and efferent motor feedback, no activity in the basal-ganglia-thalamus-cortex loop would be seen in healthy subjects, in contrast to the incomplete closing of the afferent/efferent loop and therefore an absence of the "null" signal in the case of amputees. Hence the inhibition of activity in the basal ganglia-thalamus-cortex pathway is disrupted, thereby generating an abnormal open loop functioning of the thalamocortical system and its consequent activation. This abnormal activation of the thalamocortical system, we suggest, could be the underlying cause of the conscious awareness of the phantom phenomenon.

This hypothesis is also in accordance with an emergent change of view in the functionality of the basal ganglia, from the classic view of being just part of the common motor pathway, to a more integrative, dynamic and resource-selection mechanism that participates in the sensory-motor, affective, and cognitive process related to the executive planning and selection of an action mechanism [43]. Furthermore, the conscious awareness and the subsequent sense of agency [44] which patients report to have had as they perform imagined tasks with their amputated limbs has never between contrasted with healthy subjects.

In the current study, we tested the hypothesis that the basal ganglia-thalamus-cortex pathway is disrupted in amputees, as compared to control subjects, and that this disruption is the key to the cascade of conscious awareness of the phantom limb. We contrasted between lower limb amputees and control subjects as they performed a simulated neurocognitive motor-imagery task with their phantom toes or intact toes respectively.

3. Method used

3.1. Subjects

Six unilateral lower limb amputees, 3 with left lower limb (LLL) and 3 with right lower limb (RLL) amputation (mean age 35.3, range 15-60 years, for details see Table 1), and 6 healthy controls (HC, mean age 29.16, range 20-59 years) participated in the study. All participants gave written informed consent prior to taking part in the study and the local institutional review board approved the protocol, which adhered to the Declaration of Helsinki. None of the subjects had neurological or psychiatric disorders.

	Age[1] Ctrl	Age[2] Pat	Amp[3] side	Amp[4] site	Cause of[5] Amputation	SP[6]	PLP[7]	PLS[8]
1	20	34&	RLL	TF	Traumatic	+	-	+
2	21	15	RLL	TT	Traumatic	+	-	+
3	22	44	RLL	TT	Traumatic	+	-	+
4	24	60	LLL	TT	Traumatic	+	-	+
5	29	33	LLL	TF	Traumatic	+	-	+
6	59	26	LLL	TT	Traumatic	+	-	+

Table 1. Clinical data description of controls and patients. All subjects are right handed males. [1]Column for control subjects' age. [2]Column for patients' age. [3]Three patients had right lower limb amputation and three had left lower limb amputation.[4]Site of surgery. [5]Car or train accident was main cause of amputation. [6]All the patients reported stump pain (SP), but [7]none ever had Phantom Limb Pain (PLP). [8]All patients were able to move at will their phantom toes (extension/flexion).

3.2. Experimental procedure

The experiment consisted of two parts. In the 'executed movement' condition the participants were instructed to make a flexion/extension movement with the intact (amputees) or non-dominant (HC) toes. In the condition 'imagined movements' the amputees imagined making a flexion/extension movement with the phantom toes and the HC imagined the same movement with their dominant toes. For all conditions the subjects had their eyes open. All movements or imagined movements were observed under close scrutiny by the researcher. All conditions were separate blocks of fMRI measurements with durations of 30 seconds each, separated by resting periods of 30 seconds. Each condition was repeated three times. There was no training session for either the control subjects or the amputees.

3.3. fMRI measurement

The fMRI scans were conducted with a GE 1.5 T GE LX Magnetic Resonance instrument (Milwaukee, WI, USA) using the standard quadrature headcoil. Subject's head was securely fastened in the head holder to minimize movement. Functional images were acquired with GE EPI-BOLD pulse sequence with 90° flip angle TE=60 ms, TR=3000 ms, over seven contiguous coronal sections, 8.0 mm thick with zero gap. Imaging was centered near the central gyrus. Structural images localized exactly over the same seven sections of the functional studies were obtained using a high resolution T1 weighted protocol. The activation was done in boxcar block paradigm of 30 seconds of stimulated state and 30 seconds of un-stimulated state, over a total of three blocks each.

3.4. Image analysis

All MR data was transferred to an offline workstation all images were translated into time-ordered stacks using the software MRIcro (Chris Rorden, http://www.cabiatl.com/mricro/). The experiments were analyzed subject by subject following a standard motion correction with image registration, to do a more precise alignment, since the study was acquired in coronal slices, the high resolution T1-weighted images were aligned to the T1-weighted SPM mask in MNI space, the transformations were saved and applied to the functional EPI time ordered stacks, and then the functional images were normalized to a ROI of the EPI standard provided by SPM, spatial smoothing using a Gaussian kernel of FWHM 6mm and high pass temporal filtering. Functional signal was obtained with a block model convolved with an hemodynamic response function (HRF) without time derivative correction these single subject analysis resulted in contrast maps used in the second level analysis. The second level analysis was executed to estimate group average activation using a Student–t maps limited and adjusted with $p = 0.05$ with no Volterra interactions.

4. Results

Analysis of the data was carried out for each subject individually, to see if there were statistically significant activation clusters, and then by group after combining all subjects. The average functional maps obtained revealed ipsilateral or contralateral brain activation sites, which were colored according to the tasks performed on each lower limb of all subjects: green-colored brain activation sites correspond to the right leg, while red-colored brain activation sites correspond to the left leg. Yellow-colored sites correspond to areas of overlapping activation during the performance of the tasks on each limb. The results of the three groups' brain activation sites are summarized in Table 2.

		Talairach coordinates				RIGHT		Talairach coordinates		
BRAIN REGION	BA	x	y	z		BRAIN REGION	BA	x	y	z
					Left amputee, executing right imaginary motion					
Middle Temporal Gyrus	22	-61	-37	6		Middle Temporal Gyrus	21	51	-29	-5
Paracentral Lobule	4	-10	-38	63						
Medial Frontal Gyrus	6	-6	-14	62						
Precentral Gyrus	6	-30	-20	64						
Lentiform Nucleus, Putamen	*	-26	-8	4						
					Left amputee, executing left virtual motion					
Medial Frontal Gyrus	6	-8	-11	50		Medial Frontal Gyrus	6	2	-26	64
Sub-Gyral	37	-48	-39	-5		Medial Frontal Gyrus	6	6	-9	61
Superior Temporal Gyrus	22	-59	-35	9		Substania Nigra	*	8	-24	-14
Thalamus	*	-8	-25	1		Superior Temporal Gyrus	21	48	-27	-5
Precentral Gyrus	4	-42	-11	47						
					Right amputee, executing left imaginary motion					
Superior Temporal Gyrus	22	-65	-42	15		Superior Temporal Gyrus	22	50	-4	-1
Superior Temporal Gyrus	22	-65	-18	-1		Superior Temporal Gyrus	22	50	-12	1
Postcentral Gyrus	3	-44	-17	54		Medial Frontal Gyrus	6	8	-11	50
Cingulate Gyrus	24	-8	-10	41		Middle Frontal Gyrus	6	40	-5	46
						Cingulate Gyrus	24	8	-12	37
						Thalamus	*	18	-9	13
					Right amputee, executing right virtual motion					
Precentral Gyrus	4	-12	-32	62		Superior Temporal Gyrus	22	51	-4	-3
Medial Frontal Gyrus	6	-10	-26	58						

		Talairach coordinates				RIGHT		Talairach coordinates		
BRAIN REGION	BA	x	y	z		BRAIN REGION	BA	x	y	z
Superior Temporal Gyrus	42	-63	-28	14						
Superior Temporal Gyrus	*	-63	-21	3						
Precentral Gyrus	4	-50	-12	41						
Lentiform Nucleus, Medial Globus Pallidus		-16	-10	-6						
Substania Nigra	*	-8	-10	-10						
					Control, executing left imaginary motion					
Inferior Frontal Gyrus	45	-61	20	16		Medial Frontal Gyrus	6	8	-12	71
						Medial Frontal Gyrus	6	2	-3	61
					Control, executing right imaginary motion					
Medial Frontal Gyrus	6	-2	3	51		Postcentral Gyrus	43	65	-16	21
Superior Frontal Gyrus	6	-8	-6	68						
Medial Frontal Gyrus	6	-8	1	53						
Superior Temporal Gyrus	22	-50	4	2						

BA=Brodmann Area.

Talairach coordinates: x (left[-], right[+]); y (posterior[-], anterior[+]), z (inferior[-], superior[+]). * no Brodmann area related

Table 2. Anatomical location of activation clusters during imaginary and virtual motion.

The average functional maps obtained from LLL amputee during the imaginary movement of the toes of both feet also present distinct cortical and subcortical activity. Performance of imaginary movement of the toes of the right intact toes showed activation sites bilaterally at the STG (BA 21,22), contralateral interhemispheric M1 (BA 4), contralateral SMA (BA 6), and contralateral Putamen. During the performance of imaginary movement with the left amputated toes, distinct cortical and subcortical activities were observed at the following sites: bilateral interhemispheric SMA (BA 6), bilateral STG (BA 21,22), ipsilateral M1 (BA 4), ipsilateral Subgyral (BA 37), ipsilateral Thalamus, and contralateral Substantia Nigra (figure 1,A).

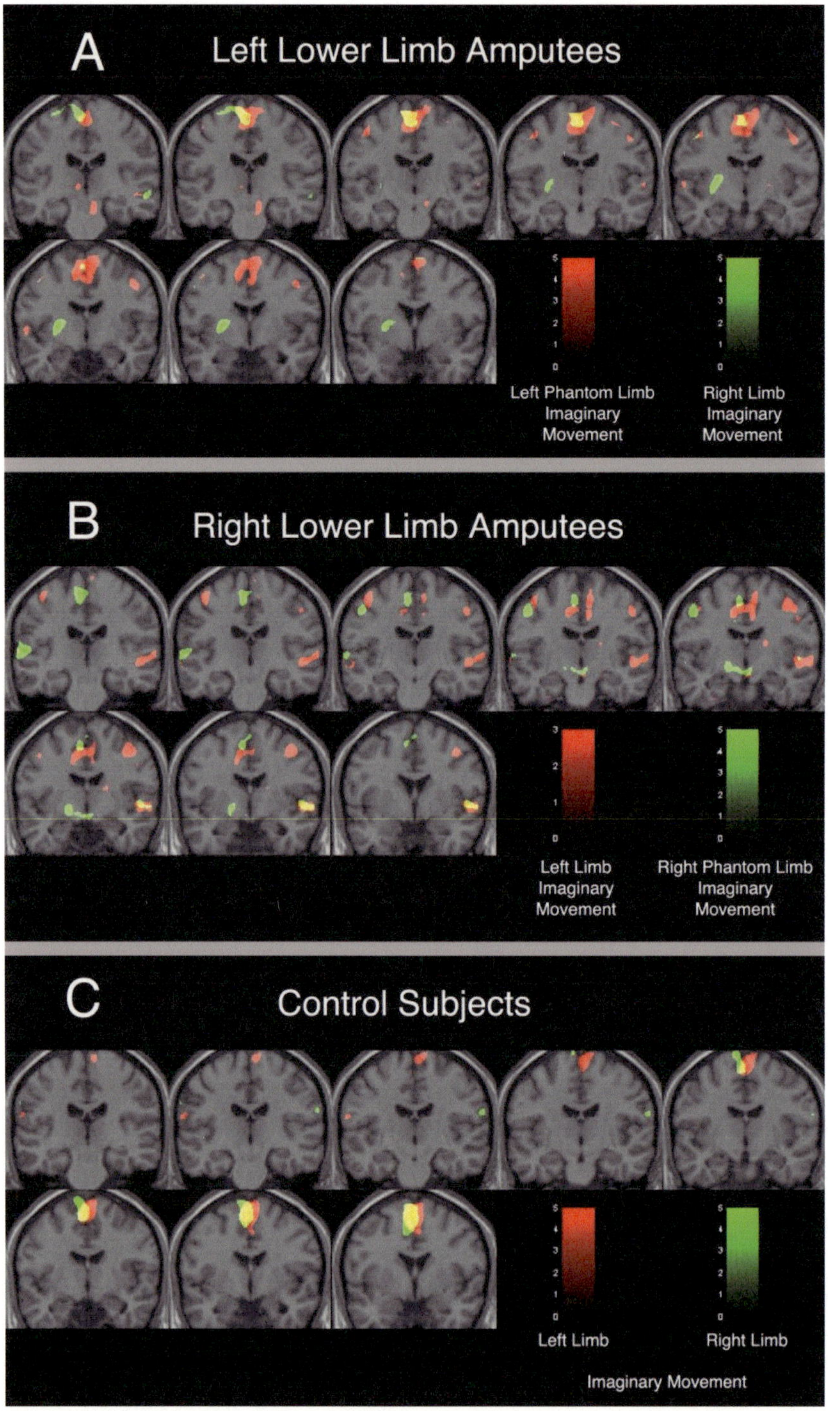

Figure 1. Average functional activation maps during imaginary movement of the right leg (in green) and left leg (in red) for A) left lower limb amputees, B) right lower limb amputees and C) control subjects. All images are presented in radiological convention.

Average functional activation maps acquired from RLL amputees during the imaginary movement of the toes of both feet depict both cortical and subcortical activities. During the performance of imaginary movement of the toes of the left intact toes, there is bilateral Temporal activity (BA 22), and bilateral Anterior Cingulate Cortex (ACC, BA 24), ipsilateral Primary Somatosensory Cortex (SI, BA 3), contralateral SMA (BA 6), and contralateral Thalamic activity, while during the performance of imaginary movement with the right amputed toes, there is a distinct activation, namely of the bilateral STG (BA 42, 22), contralateral Primary Motor Cortex (M1, BA 4), contralateral SMA (BA 6), contralateral Basal Ganglia at the Medial Globus Pallidus and at the Substantia Nigra (figure 1, B).

The average functional maps obtained from the six control subjects as they performed imaginary movement with (a) the toes of their right leg show activated contralateral sites corresponding to interhemispheric Supplementary Motor Area (SMA, BA 6), Superior Temporal Gyrus (STG, BA 22), and Ipsilateral Postcentral Gyrus (IPG, BA 43); while the performance of the same tasks with (b) the toes of their left leg, activated similar contralateral interhemispheric SMA (BA 6) and ipsilateral prefrontal (PF, BA 45) brain areas (figure 1,C).

5. Discussion

Here we compared the brain activations of imagined and executed movements of the intact toes and phantom toes in lower limb amputees, with the imagined and executed movement of the toes of healthy controls, using fMRI. Both, patients and control subject expressed that they initially had to exert greater effort in this self-generating dual process of 1) trying to resolve an apparent conflict between the simultaneous intent to move their toes and refraining from moving them or closing the sensory-motor feedback loop; and 2) locating, by means of imagery monitoring, a distant portion of the body-image, which is an attention/memory task. This sensation can be do to the increased contribution of the prefrontal cortex, in particular the dorsolateral prefrontal cortex (DLPFC), which is known to participate in motor imagery, not just in the sensory-motor integration and the attention/memory neurocognitive task with the anterior cingulate cortex, but also in a joint route with the posterior parietal cortex (PPC) during motor imagery [30,45–47]. The PPC, as a multisensory integrative cortex, plays an important role in the cognitive dynamics for spatial representation (limb-position) and movement intent, attention, working memory, and guidance of action [48,49]. As Jeannerod proposed "If motor imagery occurred with execution deliberately blocked or delayed, the representation would be protected from cancellation and would become accessible to conscious processing" [50]. Additionally, controls and amputees reported that they were consciously aware of their intact toes or, in the case of amputees, that they had the conscious perception of their phantom toes during the imaginary task. The brain activations show similarities but also differences between amputee groups during the imaginary movement tasks of their intact and amputated toes. The differences were: First, both amputee groups activate Basal Ganglia areas during the performance of the imaginary movement of the amputated toes. Second, the RLL amputee group shows more lateralized brain activation than the LLL amputee group. Third, during the imaginary movement task, the RLL amputee group seems to require a greater attention control (ACC) as they performed the imaginary movement with their left intact toes than the LLL amputee group with their right intact toes. Additionally, the brain activations observed in the amputee group during the imagery movement task of the amputated toes involved the Basal Ganglia loop (RLL amputee group = Lentiform Nucleus, Medial Globus Pallidus, and Susbtantia Nigra; LLL amputee group = Thalamus and Substantia nigra). Thus, the imagined movement task in amputees demands different circuitry subsets for its accomplishment, namely: 1) the attention/memory/guidance loop, 2) the kinesthetic imagery loop, and 3) the conflict intention loop. The computational logistics for such activity can only be carried out by means of the intracortical and cortical-subcortical loops between Thalamus and Basal Ganglia nuclei. The kinesthetic representation of an action or a planned motor intent is the combined result of a widely distributed neuronal ensemble between DLPFC, inferior frontal cortex, and the SMA [31], together with the posterior parietal cortex (PPC) and the ACC for spatial awareness, attention and multisensory integration [49,51]. It is of mayor importance to notice here that the activation of the Basal Ganglia loop was not seen during imagery movement task of the intact toes in amputees or the healthy control group. As far as the motor intent is concerned (Fig 1, B): a) in the control group, the performance of the task with the left (non-dominant) toes activated contralateral SMA (BA 6) and ipsilateral inferior frontal cortex (BA 45), while the same task with the right (dominant) toes activated contralateral SMA (BA 6), STG (BA 22), and contralateral postcentral gyrus (BA 43). The minimal brain activity found in the controls' kinesthetic representation correlates with the ensemble proposed [52,53]. b). In the RLL amputee group, in the coronal volumes (Fig 1, A), the performance of the imaginary motor intent with the left intact toes activated the bilateral ACC (BA 24), STG (BA 22), ipsilateral S1 (BA 3), and broad contralateral interhemispheric activity from SMA (BA 6) and contralateral thalamus. However, during the right imagined movement task of the amputated toes, there is bilateral activation at STG (BA 22/42), contralateral SMA (BA 6), M1 (BA 4), contralateral Lentiform Nucleus (medial globus pallidus), and Substantia Nigra. The RLL amputees' brain activity for the kinesthetic representation differed between the performance of the intact imaginary movement and the amputated imaginary movement, since Lentiform Basal Ganglia activity is only present during the amputated toes imaginary movement. c) In the coronal-volumes of the LLL amputee group (Fig 1, C) during the performance of the imaginary movement task with the right intact toes, besides a bilateral MTG (BA 21/22) activation, there is clear contralateral Lentiform Nucleus-Putamen activation, together with SMA (BA 6) and M1 (BA 4). However, during the imagery movement task with the amputated toes of the left leg, there is an ipsilateral thalamic and a Subgyral (BA 37) activation and a contralateral Substantia Nigra activation besides the large bilateral SMA (BA 6) and a bilateral MTG (BA 21/22) activations observed during the intact toes imaginary movement. The LLL amputee brain activity for the kinesthetic representation differed slightly between the performance of the imaginary movement of intact versus amputated toes, since there is Basal Ganglia activity (Putamen) during imaginary movement of the intact toes, while during amputated toes imagined movement there is Thalamic and Substantia Nigra activity. This Basal Ganglia-Thalamo-Motor-Cortex loop subserves several cortex functions, such as memory tasks, orientation in space, and the ability to change behavioral set [43,54]. In the motor imagery task, in particular in LL amputee research literature, the role of this ganglia-thalamo-motor-cortex loop has never been mentioned. In this study we set out to establish its presence using the already mentioned task in the amputee and control groups. Thus, by comparing control and amputee groups, we found that there is minimal cortical activation difference between them, however, the difference occurs in the subcortical activation of the Basal Ganglia loop, since in both, the control group and during intact toes imaginary movement of amputated subjects there is no Basal Ganglia activation, while the activation of distinct Lenticular-Substantia-Nigra-Basal-Ganglia-Thalamic loop is clear in the amputee group performing imaginary movement of the amputated toes. We thus propose that the recruitment of these Basal Ganglia plays an important role in the process of conscious awareness of a missing limb reported by amputees.

It is important to point out that we set out to find the involvement of the Basal Ganglia-Thalamic-Motor-Cortex loop by means of this motor imagery task, as part of our hypothesis that the amputee can and does move the phantom limbs at will, this, do to his framework of body awareness as part of a self-related neurocognitive experience that can be as diverse as the perceiving of size, shape, posture, itch, touch, pressure, vibration, temperature, 'electric' sensations and prosthesis embodiment and has been well documented [20]. Similar to Ramachandran´s "null" hypothesis [17] we think that the interruption of the thalamic afferences/efferences may explain the persistence of an open loop functioning of the thalamocortical system and its consequent activation, which is a key factor to the cascade of conscious awareness and stability of the phantom phenomenon. This open loop functioning of the thalamocortical system is revealed in the present study by the increased blood oxygen level-dependent (BOLD) signal in the Basal Ganglia-Thalamic-Motor-Cortex loop pathway during imaginary movement of the amputated toes. Thus, supporting our hypothesis of the abnormal closed-loop functioning of the thalamocortical system as underlying the phantom phenomenon.

6. Conclusion

To conclude, we have put forward evidence of amputee patients' indirect responses to PL experiences for an objective evaluation that suggests that the conscious awareness of a phantom limb emerges from both the reduction in afferent information and the higher-level brain reorganization of the cognitive representations of the amputee's own body. We based our assumptions on the hypothesis that the thalamocortical loop is closed in healthy subjects, which enable them to distinguish an imaginary movement as actually being just imagined. This, do to the feedback received from intact peripheric (efferent/afferent) information pathways. The evidence shown here thus suggests that this abnormal open loop of the basal-ganglia-thalamocortical system underlies the conscious awareness of the phantom limb. The current approach further suggests that the basal ganglia within this basal-ganglia-thalamocortical system loop play a crucial and complex integration of afferent and efferent information processing. Furthermore, this integration creates the conscious awareness of the self and is in line with the internal model theory of motor control [15] where inverse and forward models of information processing interact continuously and reciprocally. The inverse model component in the motor system providing the motor commands necessary to achieve a desired consequence of an action, specified by higher-level goals and the forward model predicting the sensory consequences of each of these motor programs to be executed. Accordingly, whenever a motor program is issued, an efference copy is produced in parallel and an accurate prediction of the sensory consequences expected after the execution of the program, which in turn informs the inverse program of the actual state of the self and closing the loop for the next command. With this normally closed loop, the integration of the self is achieved and a normal body ownership and awareness is crated which is necessary to create the autobiographical experience of self.

Glossary of terms

Bottom-up: direction of information flow from the periphery (i.e. sensory cells or mechanoreceptors) to the central nervous system.
Top-down: information flow from central nervous system toward peripheral effector cells (i.e. muscles).
Efferent: Conveying away from the central nervous system
Afferent: Conveying towards a central nervous system
Phantom limb: is the sensation that an amputated or missing limb is still attached to the body
Somatosensory system: sensory system composed of the receptors and processing centers to produce the sensory modalities such as touch, temperature, proprioception (body position), and nociception (pain).
Proprioception: sensory modality that processes the body position
Ipsilateral: same side of the body
Contralateral: other side of the body

Author details

Clemens C.C. Bauer*, Erick H. Pasaye and Fernando A. Barrios
Neurobiology Institute, Universidad Autónoma de México, Querétaro, México

Juan I. Romero-Romo
Querétaro General Hospital, SESEQ; Queretaro, Mexico

Acknowledgement

We want to thank Dr. Perla Salgado and Dr. Rafael Rojas form the Imaging Department of The ABC Medical Center, Mexico City. This work was partially supported by CONACyT R31162-A, and a Doctoral Schollarship from CONACyT México and the Doctoral Program in Biomedical Sciences in the Institute of Neurobiology, Universidad Nacional Autónoma de

---

* Corresponding Author

México for CCCB and EHP. We thank Leopoldo Gonzalez-Santos, Juan J. Ortiz for their technical support.

7. References

[1] Draganski B, Kherif F, Klöppel S, Cook PA, Alexander DC, Parker GJM, et al. (2008) Evidence for Segregated and Integrative Connectivity Patterns in the Human Basal Ganglia. Journal of Neuroscience. 9;28(28):7143–52.

[2] Alexander GE, DeLong MR, Strick PL. (1986) Parallel organization of functionally segregated circuits linking basal ganglia and cortex. Annual Review of Neuroscience. 9(1):357–81.

[3] Lotze M, Montoya P, Erb M, Hülsmann E, Flor H, Klose U, et al. (1999) Activation of cortical and cerebellar motor areas during executed and imagined hand movements: an fMRI study. Journal of Cognitive Neuroscience. 11(5):491–501.

[4] Lorey B, Bischoff M, Pilgramm S, Stark R, Munzert J, Zentgraf K. (2009) The embodied nature of motor imagery: the influence of posture and perspective. Experimental Brain research. 194(2):233–43.

[5] Mizumori SJ., Puryear CB, Martig AK. (2009) Basal ganglia contributions to adaptive navigation. Behavioural brain Research. 199(1):32–42.

[6] Kotz SA, Schwartze M, Schmidt-Kassow M. (2009) Non-motor basal ganglia functions: a review and proposal for a model of sensory predictability in auditory language perception. Cortex. 45(8):982–90.

[7] Bernsz S, Sejnowskil TJ. (2010) How the basal ganglia make decisions. Available: http://papers.cnl.salk.edu/PDFs/How%20the%20Basal%20Ganglia%20Make%20Decisions%201996-2876.pdf. Accesed 2012 March

[8] van Schouwenburg MR, den Ouden HE., Cools R. (2010) The human basal ganglia modulate frontal-posterior connectivity during attention shifting. The Journal of Neuroscience. 30(29):9910–8.

[9] Provost JS, Petrides M, Monchi O. (2010) Dissociating the role of the caudate nucleus and dorsolateral prefrontal cortex in the monitoring of events within human working memory. European Journal of Neuroscience. 32(5):873–80.

[10] Friederici AD, Kotz SA. (2003) The brain basis of syntactic processes: functional imaging and lesion studies. Neuroimage. 20:S8–S17.

[11] Booth JR, Wood L, Lu D, Houk JC, Bitan T. (2007) The role of the basal ganglia and cerebellum in language processing. Brain Research. 1133:136–44.

[12] Middleton FA, Strick PL. (2000) Basal ganglia and cerebellar loops: motor and cognitive circuits. Brain Research Reviews. 31(2-3):236–50.

[13] Kircher TTJ, Leube DT. (2003) Self-consciousness, self-agency, and schizophrenia. Consciousness and Cognition. 12(4):656–69.

[14] Lycan WG. (1996) Consciousness and Experience. A Bradford Book.

[15] Frith CD, Wolpert DM. (2000) Abnormalities in the awareness and control of action. Philosophical Transactions of the Royal Society of London. Series B: Biological Sciences. 355(1404):1771–88.

[16] Holst E, (1950) Mittelstaedt H. Das reafferenzprinzip. Naturwissenschaften. 37(20):464–76.

[17] Ramachandran VS, Brang D. (2009) Sensations evoked in patients with amputation from watching an individual whose corresponding intact limb is being touched. Archives of Neurology. 66(10):1281.

[18] Kircher T, David AS. (2003) The self in neuroscience and psychiatry. Cambridge Univ Pr.

[19] Serino A, Haggard P. (2010) Touch and the body. Neuroscience & Biobehavioral Reviews. 34(2):224–36.

[20] Giummarra MJ, Georgiou-Karistianis N, Nicholls ME., Gibson SJ, Chou M, Bradshaw JL. (2010) Corporeal awareness and proprioceptive sense of the phantom. British Journal of Psychology. 101(4):791–808.

[21] Hunter JP, Katz J, Davis KD.(2008) Stability of phantom limb phenomena after upper limb amputation: a longitudinal study. Neuroscience. 156(4):939–49.

[22] Halligan PW. (2002) Phantom limbs: the body in mind. Cognitive Neuropsychiatry. 7(3):251–69.

[23] Ramachandran VS, Hirstein W. (1998) The perception of phantom limbs. The DO Hebb lecture. Brain. 121(9):1603.

[24] Arzy S, Thut G, Mohr C, Michel CM, Blanke O. (2006) Neural basis of embodiment: distinct contributions of temporoparietal junction and extrastriate body area. The Journal of Neuroscience. 26(31):8074.

[25] Schreiber A, Ball T, Kristeva-Feige R, Mergner T, Feige B, Scheremet R, et al. (1998) Primary and Secondary Motor Areas in fMRI and EEG. Available: http://cds. ismrm.org/ismrm-1998/PDF6/p1568.pdf. Accessed 2012 March

[26] Stippich C, Freitag P, Kassubek J, Sörös P, Kamada K, Kober H, et al. (1998) Motor, somatosensory and auditory cortex localization by fMRI and MEG. Neuroreport. 9(9):1953.

[27] Flor H, Elbert T, Mühlnickel W, Pantev C, Wienbruch C, Taub E. (1998) Cortical reorganization and phantom phenomena in congenital and traumatic upper-extremity amputees. Experimental Brain Research. 119(2):205–12.

[28] Condés-Lara M, Barrios FA, Romo JR, Rojas R, Salgado P, Sánchez-Cortazar J. (2000) Brain somatic representation of phantom and intact limb: a fMRI study case report. European Journal of Pain. 4(3):239–45.

[29] Nitschke MF, Kleinschmidt A, Wessel K, Frahm J. (1996) Somatotopic motor representation in the human anterior cerebellum. A high-resolution functional MRI study. Brain: Brain (1996) 119 (3): 1023-1029. doi: 10.1093/brain/119.3.1023.

[30] Ersland L, Rosén G, Lundervold A, Smievoll AI, Tillung T, Sundberg H. (1996) Phantom limb imaginary fingertapping causes primary motor cortex activation: an fMRI study. Neuroreport. 8(1):207.

[31] Jeannerod M, Frak V. (1999) Mental imaging of motor activity in humans. Current Opinion in Neurobiology. 9(6):735–9.

[32] Ganis G, Thompson WL, Kosslyn SM. (2004) Brain areas underlying visual mental imagery and visual perception: an fMRI study. Cognitive Brain Research. 20(2):226–41.

[33] Lotze M, Flor H, Grodd W, Larbig W, Birbaumer N. (2001) Phantom movements and pain An fMRI study in upper limb amputees. Brain. 124(11):2268.
[34] Diers M, Christmann C, Koeppe C, Ruf M, Flor H. (2010) Mirrored, imagined and executed movements differentially activate sensorimotor cortex in amputees with and without phantom limb pain. Pain. 149(2):296–304.
[35] Pasaye E, Gutiérrez R, Alcauter S, Mercadillo R, Aguilar-Castañeda E, de Iturbe M, et al. (2010) Event-Related Functional Magnetic Resonance Images During the Perception of Phantom Limb; a Brushing Task. The Neuroradiology Journal. 23:665–70.
[36] Pick A. Zur Pathologie des Bewußtseins vom eigenen Körper. (1915) Ein Beitrag aus der Kriegsmedizin. Neurologisches Zentralblatt. 34:257–65.
[37] Levine DN. (1990) Unawareness of visual and sensorimotor defects: A hypothesis. Brain and Cognition. 13(2):233–81.
[38] Ramachandran VS, Hirstein W. (1998) The perception of phantom limbs. The DO Hebb lecture. Brain. 121(9):1603.
[39] Heilman KM. (1991) Anosognosia: possible neuropsychological mechanisms. In Prigatano, G. P., & Schacter, D. L. (1991). Awareness of deficit after brain injury: Clinical and theoretical issues. pp 53- 62. Oxford University Press, USA.
[40] Gallese V. (2007) The "conscious" dorsal stream: embodied simulation and its role in space and action conscious awareness. Psyche. 13(1):1–20.
[41] Staub F, Bogousslavsky J, Maeder P, Maeder-Ingvar M, Fornari E, Ghika J, et al. (2006) Intentional motor phantom limb syndrome. Neurology. 67(12):2140–6.
[42] Fitzgibbon BM, Giummarra MJ, Georgiou-Karistianis N, Enticott PG, Bradshaw JL. (2010) Shared pain: from empathy to synaesthesia. Neuroscience & Biobehavioral Reviews. 34(4):500–12.
[43] Gurney K, Prescott TJ, Wickens JR, Redgrave P. (2004) Computational models of the basal ganglia: from robots to membranes. Trends in Neurosciences. 27(8):453–9.
[44] Ramachandran VS. (1993) Behavioral and magnetoencephalographic correlates of plasticity in the adult human brain. Proceedings of the National Academy of Sciences of the United States of America. 90(22):10413.
[45] Decety J, Perani D, Jeannerod M, Bettinardi V, Tadary B, Woods R, et al. (1994) Mapping motor representations with positron emission tomography. Nature. 371, 600-602
[46] Stephan KM, Fink GR, Passingham RE, Silbersweig D, Ceballos-Baumann AO, Frith CD, et al. (1995) Functional anatomy of the mental representation of upper extremity movements in healthy subjects. Journal of Neurophysiology. 73(1):373–86.
[47] Boussaoud D. (2001) Attention versus intention in the primate premotor cortex. Neuroimage. 14(1):S40–S45.
[48] Culham JC, Kanwisher NG. (2001) Neuroimaging of cognitive functions in human parietal cortex. Current Opinion in Neurobiology. 11(2):157–63.
[49] Andersen RA, Buneo CA. (2002) Intentional maps in posterior parietal cortex. Annual Review of Neuroscience. 25(1):189–220.
[50] Jeannerod M. (1994) The representing brain: Neural correlates of motor intention and imagery. Behavioral and Brain Sciences. 17(02):187–202.

[51] Crammond DJ. (1997) Motor imagery: never in your wildest dream. Trends in Neurosciences. 20(2):54.
[52] Jackson PL, Decety J. (2004) Motor cognition: a new paradigm to study self-other interactions. Current Opinion in Neurobiology. 14(2):259–63.
[53] Jeannerod M, Decety J. (1995) Mental motor imagery: a window into the representational stages of action. Current Opinion in Neurobiology. 5(6):727–32.
[54] Yang TT, Gallen CC, Ramachandran VS, Cobb S. (1994) Noninvasive detection of cerebral plasticity in adult human somatosensory cortex. Neuroreport: An International Journal for the Rapid Communication of Research in Neuroscience.Vol 5(6), 701-704.

Chapter 5

Organization of Two Cortico–Basal Ganglia Loop Circuits That Arise from Distinct Sectors of the Monkey Dorsal Premotor Cortex

Masahiko Takada, Eiji Hoshi, Yosuke Saga, Ken-ichi Inoue, Shigehiro Miyachi, Nobuhiko Hatanaka, Masahiko Inase and Atsushi Nambu

Additional information is available at the end of the chapter

http://dx.doi.org/10.5772/54822

1. Introduction

The importance of loop circuits linking the frontal cortex and the basal ganglia has constantly been highlighted in the performance of various motor schemes [1-4]. These cortico–basal ganglia loop circuits originate from anatomically and functionally diverse motor-related areas, which include the primary motor cortex (MI), the supplementary motor area (SMA), and the premotor cortex (PM). Two opposing mechanisms are possible for the processing of motor information in the cortico–basal ganglia loops. One is "information funneling" in which inputs from multiple motor-related areas are highly concentrated in common territories of the basal ganglia. The other is "parallel processing" in which inputs from distinct motor-related areas are topographically distributed to individual territories of the basal ganglia. For understanding the mode of motor information processing in the basal ganglia, it is crucial to investigate which mechanism organizes the projections from the frontal motor-related areas to the input stations of the basal ganglia, the striatum and the subthalamic nucleus (STN).

According to several physiological studies [5-8], it has been revealed that the caudal aspect of the dorsal premotor cortex (F2; see [9,10]) in area 6 of macaque monkeys plays a crucial role in the planning and execution of arm movements, and that there is certain functional specialization between the caudal sector of F2 (F2c), located ventral to the superior precentral dimple, and the rostral sector of F2 (F2r), located dorsal to the genu of the arcuate sulcus. Since our prior work demonstrates that F2c and F2r receive largely segregated inputs from the cerebellum [11], it is of great interest to explore the organization of cortico–basal ganglia loop circuits that arise from F2c and F2r.

In this chapter, we first summarize a series of our previous anatomical studies about the mode of information processing in the basal ganglia based on the distribution patterns of corticostriatal and corticosubthalamic inputs from the frontal motor-related areas of macaque monkeys, including the PM [12-18]. The overall results indicate that the corticostriatal and corticosubthalamic inputs from the motor-related areas are orderly arranged according to segregation versus overlap rules. We then introduce the data of our recent work concerning the organization of multisynaptic pathways that connect the basal ganglia with F2. In this study, we investigated the distributions of cells of origin in the basal ganglia of multisynaptic inputs to F2c and F2r [19]. Employing retrograde transsynaptic transport of rabies virus, we have demonstrated that neuronal populations giving rise to the projections to F2c and F2r are substantially segregated in the internal segment of the globus pallidus (GPi) and the substantia nigra pars reticulata (SNr) (i.e., the output stations of the basal ganglia), whereas intermingling rather than segregation governs for the other basal ganglia components, involving the external segment of the globus pallidus (GPe), STN, and the striatum (i.e., the input stations of the basal ganglia). This suggests that the loop circuits linking F2 and the basal ganglia may possess a common convergent window at the input stage and constitute parallel divergent channels at the output stage. The major part the present experiments was carried out at the Tokyo Metropolitan Institute for Neuroscience, Tokyo Metropolitan Organization for Medical Research. The experimental protocol was approved by the Animal Care and Use Committee of the Tokyo Metropolitan Institute for Neuroscience, and all experiments were conducted in accordance with the Guidelines for the Care and Use of Animals (Tokyo Metropolitan Institute for Neuroscience, 2000).

2. Organization of corticostriatal and corticosubthalamic inputs

In a series of our previous anatomical studies, we have analyzed the distribution patterns of corticostriatal and corticosubthalamic inputs from the frontal motor-related areas of macaque monkeys [12-18]. The frontal motor-related areas that we have examined widely include the MI, SMA, dorsal and ventral divisions of the PM (PMd and PMv), presupplementary motor area (pre-SMA), and rostral and caudal divisions of the cingulate motor area (CMAr and CMAc). In our studies, we initially performed intracortical microstimulation to map these areas. Then, different anterograde tracers were injected separately into somatotopically corresponding regions of given areas; the forelimb regions were tested except for the MI and SMA). The overall results indicate that corticostriatal and corticosubthalamic input zones from the frontal motor-related areas are orderly distributed in a topographical fashion, but display complex patterns of segregation versus overlap of one another (Figs. 1, 2).

With respect to the corticostriatal inputs from the MI and SMA, dense input zones from the MI are located predominantly in the lateral aspect of the caudal putamen, whereas those from the SMA are in the medial aspect. On the other hand, corticostriatal inputs from the PMd and PMv are distributed mainly in the dorsomedial sector of the putamen, although these two input zones are virtually devoid of overlap. Thus, the corticostriatal input zones from the MI and SMA were considerably segregated though partly overlapped in the mediolateral central aspect of the putamen, while the corticostriatal input zones from the

PMd and PMv largely overlap that from the SMA, but not from the MI (Fig. 1; see also [14,15]). In addition, the corticostriatal input zone from the pre-SMA is located primarily in the striatal cell bridges and their neighboring regions of the caudate nucleus and the putamen, thus indicating that the corticostriatal input from the pre-SMA is spatially separate from those from the MI, SMA, and PMd/PMv (Fig. 1; see also [17]). As for the CMAr and CMAc, corticostriatal inputs from the CMAr and CMAc are located within the rostral striatum, with the highest density in the striatal cell bridge region or the ventrolateral portion of the putamen, respectively. There is no substantial overlap between these input zones. The corticostriatal input zone from the CMAr considerably overlaps that from the pre-SMA, while the input zone from the CMAc displays a large overlap with that from the MI (Fig. 1; see also [16]). Moreover, it has also shown that the rostral aspect of the PMd (F7; see [9,10]) projects predominantly to the striatal cell bridge region [18].

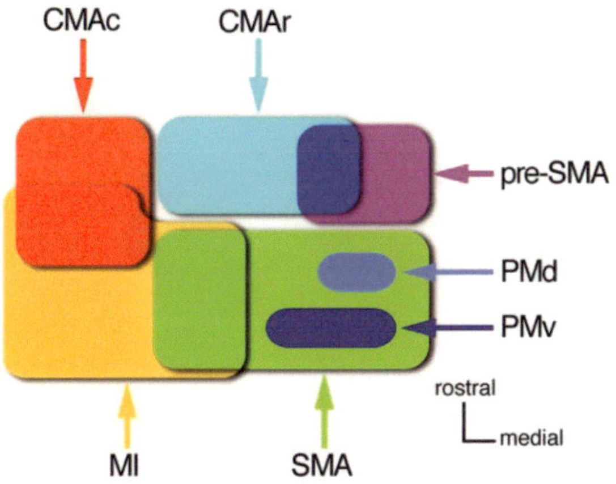

Figure 1. Summary diagram showing the organization of corticostriatal input zones in the putamen that arise from the frontal motor-related areas. These input zones are orderly distributed in a topographical fashion, but display complex patterns of segregation and overlap.

The overall pattern of corticosubthalamic input distributions is essentially the same as that of corticostriatal input distributions. The corticosubthalamic input zones from the MI and CMAc are located mainly within the lateral aspect of the STN, thereby leading to a large overlap of the two input zones. On the other hand, the major input zones from the SMA, pre-SMA, PMd, PMv, and CMAr within the medial aspect of the STN where a varying degree of overlaps are apparent between the input zones (Fig. 2; see also [12,13,16,17].

In terms of the somatotopical representation, the corticostriatal input zones from regions of the frontal motor-related areas (i.e., the MI, SMA, and PM) representing the hindlimb, forelimb, and orofacial part are, in this order, arranged from dorsal to ventral within the putamen (Fig. 3; see also [14]). A similar pattern is most likely to organize the somatotopical arrangement of cortical motor inputs within the GPe and GPi (Fig. 3). Of particular interest is that dual sets of body part representations underlie the somatotopical arrangement in the STN. Somatotopical representations in the lateral part of the STN are arranged from medial to lateral in the order of the hindlimb, forelimb, and orofacial part. By contrast, these body parts in the medial counterpart are represented mediolaterally in the inverse order, as though reflecting a "mirror image" against the somatotopical arrangement in the lateral STN (Fig. 3; see also [12]).

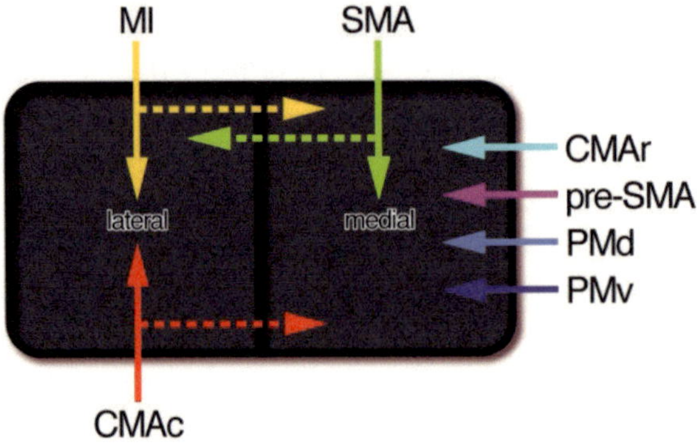

Figure 2. Summary diagram showing the organization of corticosubthalamic input zones from the frontal motor-related areas. Broken arrows represent minor projections.

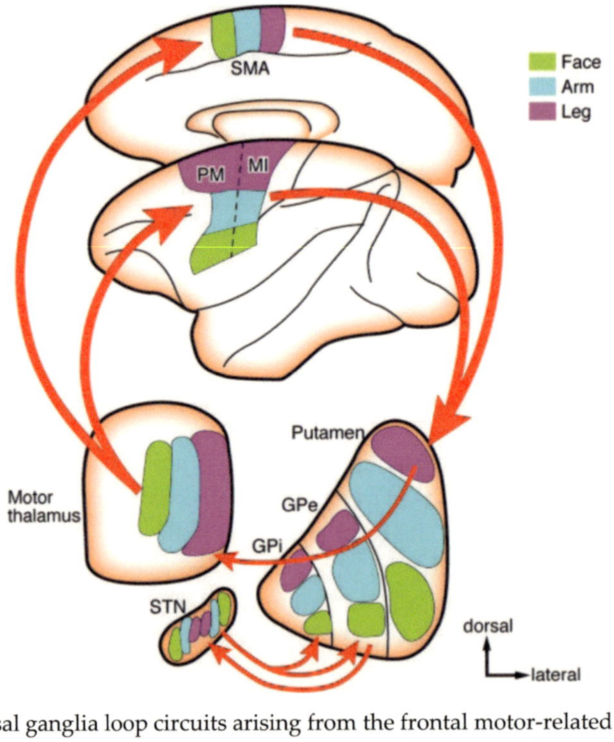

Figure 3. Cortico–basal ganglia loop circuits arising from the frontal motor-related areas (i.e., the MI, SMA, and PM) in terms of the somatotopical representation. Corticostriatal input zones from regions of representing the hindlimb, forelimb, and orofacial part are, in this order, arranged from dorsal to ventral within the putamen and GPe/GPi. In the STN, there exist dual sets of body part representations. Somatotopical representations in the lateral STN are arranged from medial to lateral in the order of the hindlimb, forelimb, and orofacial part, whereas the medial STN exhibits a mediolaterally reversed pattern of the representations, thereby reflecting a "mirror image" against the somatotopical arrangement in the lateral STN.

3. Organization of multisynaptic pathways linking F2 and the basal ganglia

3.1. Rabies injections

Multiple injections of rabies virus were made into F2c and F2r in the PMd (Fig. 4). The injection sites were determined according to the results of our previous electrophysiological work in which we demonstrated that the neuronal response properties involved in planning and executing reaching movements differed in F2r and F2c [20]. This rostrocaudal segregation is consistent with the classification schema that emerged in previous studies [10,21,22]. The rabies injections were carried out lateral to the superior precentral dimple for the F2c procedure (Fig. 4B). For the F2r procedure, on the other hand, the rabies injections were done around the genu of the arcuate sulcus (Fig. 4C).

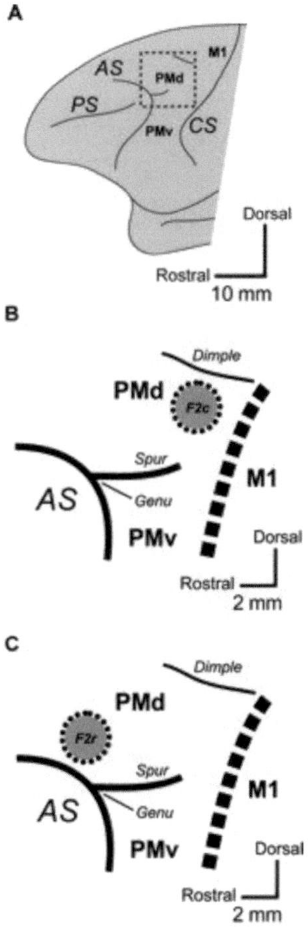

Figure 4. Locations of the injection sites in F2c and F2r. (A) Diagram illustrating the macaque lateral frontal lobe. The rectangular area drawn with broken lines in (A) is enlarged in (B) and (C). (B,C) Injection sites of rabies virus in F2c (B) and F2r (C). In (B) and (C), the border between the PMd/PMv and the MI is represented with the broken line. AS, arcuate sulcus; CS, central sulcus; Dimple, superior precentral dimple; Genu, genu of the AS; PS, principal sulcus; Spur, spur of the AS.

3.2. Origins of basal ganglia inputs to F2c and F2r

Three days after the rabies injection into F2c or F2r, a number of labeled neurons were observed in the GPi and SNr. These neurons are considered to send outputs to F2c or F2r via the ventral nuclei or mediodorsal nucleus of the thalamus. No labeled neurons were found in the GPe at this stage, indicating that only the second-order neuron labeling occurred at the 3-day postinjection period.

The distribution of labeled neurons observed in the GPi after the F2c injection differed from that observed after the F2r injection (Fig. 5). Two-dimensional density maps of the GPi were prepared to separately represent the labeling patterns in outer and inner portions (Fig. 5A). These maps showed that the distributions of GPi neurons projecting to F2c and F2r were segregated in both portions, each of which received input from the striatum [23]. After the F2c injection, the labeled neurons were distributed broadly in the ventral part of the GPi at its caudal level (Fig. 5B). By contrast, the labeled neurons after the F2r injection were located in the dorsal part of the GPi at its rostocaudal middle level (Fig. 5C).

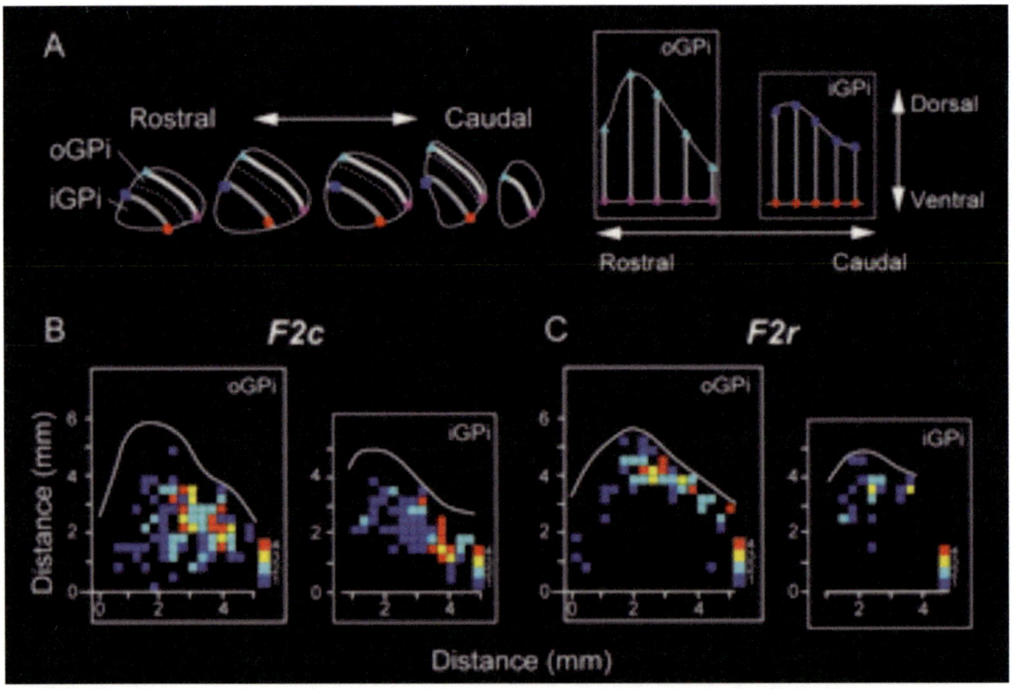

Figure 5. Density maps of GPi neuron labeling after rabies injections into F2c and F2r. (A) Procedures to construct two-dimensional density maps of the GPi. The unfolding process started with drawing lines through the center of the outer (oGPi) and inner (iGPi) portions of the GPi (left). The reference points were placed at the bottom (specified by pink stars or red circles) and the top (specified by cyan triangles or blue squares) of the GPi. The position of each labeled neuron was projected onto the central line. Then, each line through the nucleus was aligned on the ventral edge of the GPi (right). The GPi was divided into 300 μm x 300 μm bins. (B) Density maps of oGPi and iGPi neuron labeling after F2c injection. (C) Density maps of oGPi and iGPi neuron labeling after F2r injection. The number of labeled neurons in each bin was counted and color-coded.

The rabies injections into F2c and F2r resulted in different distributions of neuronal labeling in the SNr. After the F2c injection, labeled neurons in the SNr were found in the central part through the caudal half of the SNr. After the F2r injection, on the other hand, labeled neurons were distributed primarily throughout the rostral half of the SNr (data not shown).

By extending the postinjection period to 4 days, we detected neuronal labeling in the GPe, STN, and striatum. In the GPe, labeled neurons were widely distributed over the nucleus following the F2c injection, whereas they occupied a more restricted area following the F2r injection (Fig. 6). To compare the two distribution patterns in detail, two-dimensional density maps of the GPe were prepared to depict the results from the F2c and F2r injections (Fig. 6A). In the F2r injection case, the labeled neurons were located only in the rostral and dorsal portions of the GPe (Fig. 6C), while those in the F2c injection case were found not only in the rostral and dorsal portions, but also in the caudal and ventral portions of the GPe (Fig. 6B). These data indicated that the area in which GPe neurons projected trisynaptically to F2r was included within the area in which GPe neurons projected to F2c.

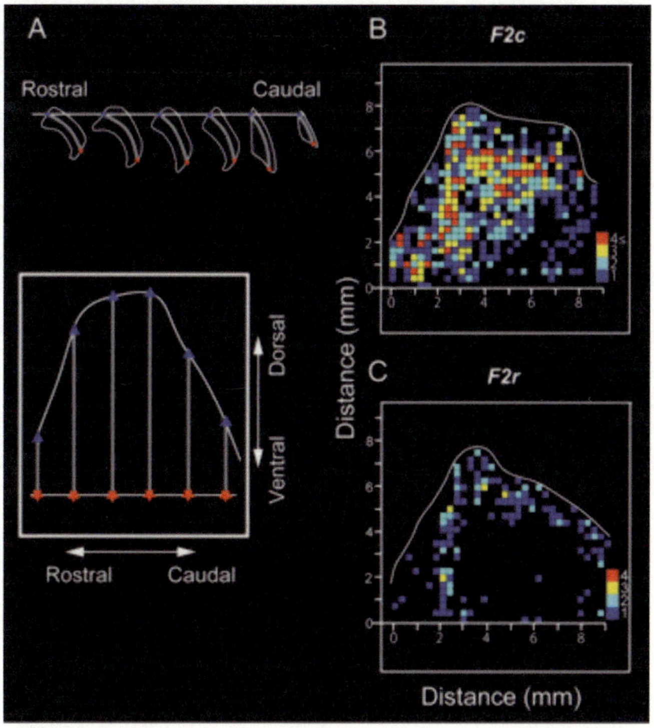

Figure 6. Density maps of GPe neuron labeling after rabies injections into F2c and F2r. (A) Procedures to construct two-dimensional density maps of the GPe. The unfolding process started with drawing lines through the center of the GPe (top). The reference points were placed at the bottom (specified by red stars) and the top (specified by blue triangles) of the GPe. The position of each labeled neuron was projected onto the central line. Then, each line through the nucleus was aligned on the ventral edge of the GPe (bottom). The GPe was divided into 300 µm x 300 µm bins. (B) Density map of GPe neuron labeling after F2c injection. (C) Density map of GPe neuron labeling after F2r injection. The number of labeled neurons in each bin was counted and color-coded.

In Figure 7, density maps of neuronal labeling in the STN are shown. After the F2r injection, labeled neurons were located primarily in the ventral aspect (Fig. 7, lower row), whereas the area of rabies labeling after the F2c injection expanded more dorsally (Fig. 7, upper row).

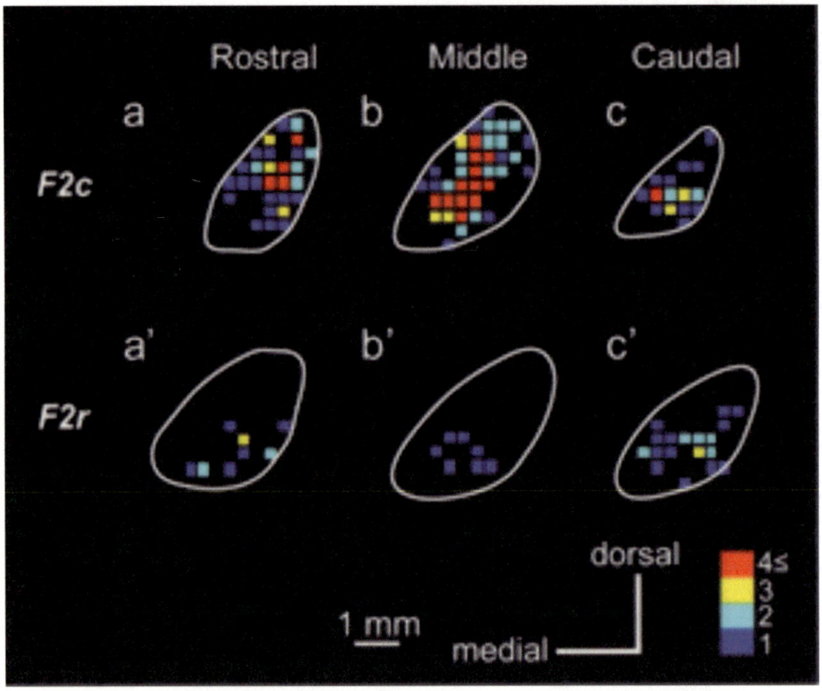

Figure 7. Distributions of STN neuron labeling after rabies injections into F2c and F2r. Three equidistant coronal sections are arranged rostrocaudally in a-c (after F2c injection) and a′-c′ (after F2r injection). The STN was divided into 300 μm x 300 μm bins. The number of labeled neurons in each bin was counted and color-coded.

Large numbers of labeled neurons were observed in the striatum. Following each injection, the labeled neurons were widely distributed in the striatal cell bridges and their neighboring regions of the caudate nucleus and the putamen (Fig. 8). In addition, dense neuron labeling was seen in the ventral striatum (Fig. 8).

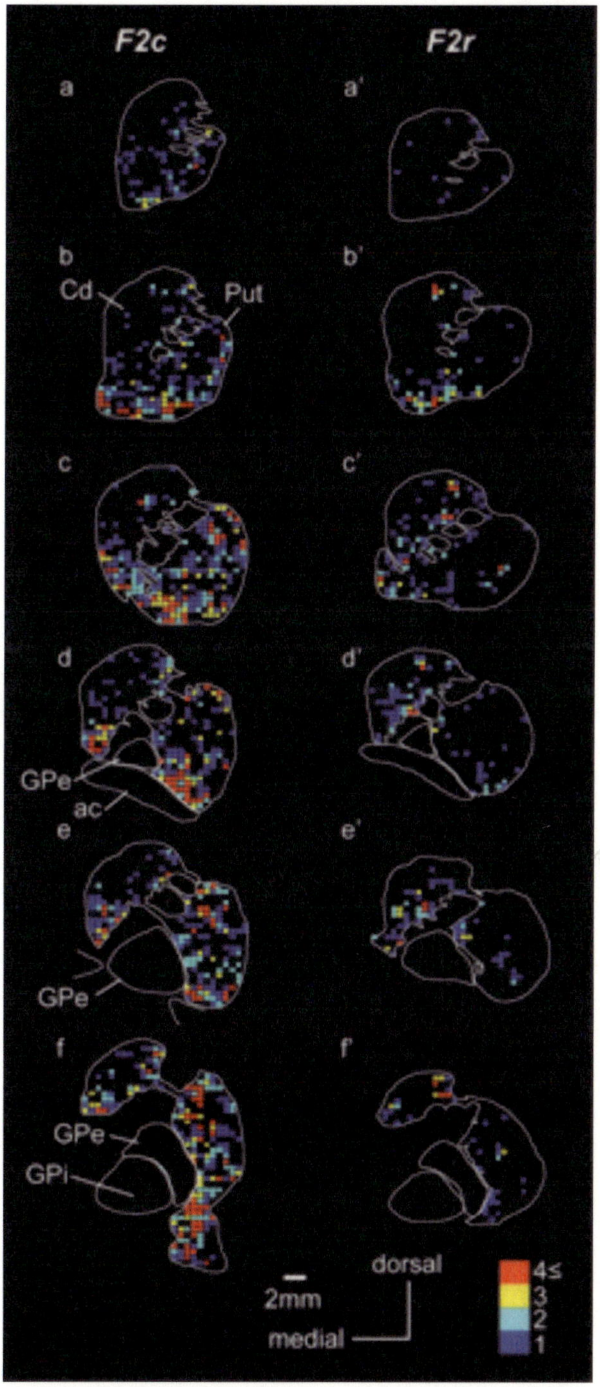

Figure 8. Distributions of striatal neuron labeling after rabies injections into F2c and F2r. Six equidistant coronal sections are arranged rostrocaudally in a-f (after F2c injection) and a'-f' (after F2r injection). The striatum was divided into 500 μm x 500 μm bins. The number of labeled neurons in each bin was counted and color-coded. ac, anterior commissure; Cd, caudate nucleus; Put, putamen.

4. Conclusion

Here, we propose that two separate channels, each of which projects multisynaptically to F2c and F2r, may be operated in the output stations of the basal ganglia (i.e., the GPi and SNr), although segregation may be obscured in the input station (i.e., the striatum) where neurons projecting multisynaptically to F2c and F2r intermingle (Fig. 9). This indicates that each of the two parallel loops (i.e., the F2c-basal ganglia loop and the F2r-basal ganglia loop)

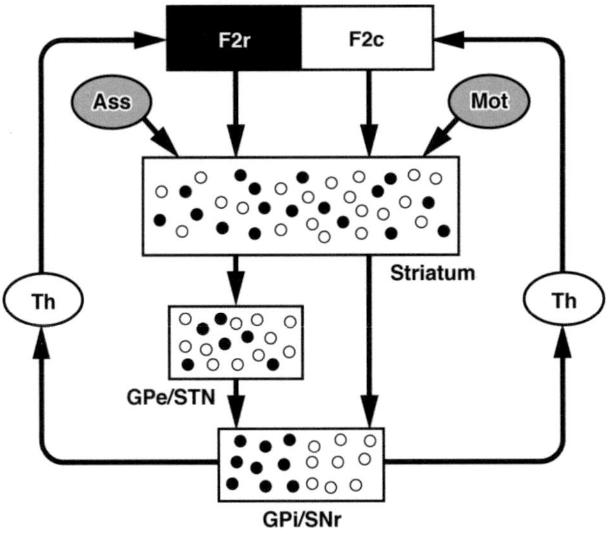

Figure 9. Schematic diagram showing the distribution patterns of cells of origin in the basal ganglia of multisynaptic inputs to F2c and F2r. In the striatum, GPe/STN, and GPi/SNr, open and filled circles indicate neurons projecting multisynaptically to F2c and F2r, respectively. In the output stations of the basal ganglia (i.e., GPi/SNr), the cells of origin of multisynaptic projections to F2c and F2r are basically segregated. On the other hand, intermingling rather than segregation is prominent for the other basal ganglia components, including the input station (i.e., striatum). Note that in the GPe/STN that connects the input and output stations, the F2r territory tends to be included within the F2c territory (see the text for detail). Ass, association cortical areas such as the prefrontal cortex; Mot, motor cortical areas such as the MI and SMA; Th, thalamus.

collects diverse inputs from the motor and association territories with which F2c and F2r are cortically interconnected. Given that individual neurons in the GPi and SNr have widespread dendritic trees [24,25], these structures may consist of zones where diverse inputs are sorted and integrated, which allows each structure to send outputs to F2c and F2r separately. On the other hand, the distribution pattern of neurons in the GPe and STN that project multisynaptically to F2c and F2r differs from that of neurons in the GPi and SNr; the F2r territory seems to be included within the F2c territory in the GPe and STN. This suggests that the mode of information processing in the GPe and STN may be distinct from that in the GPi and SNr. Together with a previous notion that there is the precise network architecture in each component of the basal ganglia [26-28], our overall results will provide a novel framework for understanding the mode of information processing in the cortico–basal ganglia loop circuits.

By analyzing the network linking F2 and the cerebellum, we have revealed that the cells of origin in the cerebellum of multisynaptic projections to F2c and F2r are segregated at the output station (i.e., the deep cerebellar nuclei), whereas both integration and segregation are evident at the input station (i.e., the cerebellar cortex) [11]. The networks connecting the basal ganglia/cerebellum with F2 may be governed by a common rule organizing the segregation at the output stage and the intermingling rather than the segregation at the input stage.

Author details

Masahiko Takada* and Ken-ichi Inoue
Systems Neuroscience Section, Primate Research Institute, Kyoto University, Inuyama, Japan

Masahiko Takada, Eiji Hoshi and Atsushi Nambu
Japan Science and Technology Agency, CREST, Tokyo, Japan

Eiji Hoshi and Yosuke Saga
Frontal Lobe Project, Tokyo Metropolitan Institute of Medical Science, Tokyo, Japan

Shigehiro Miyachi
Cognitive Neuroscience Section, Primate Research Institute, Kyoto University, Inuyama, Japan

Nobuhiko Hatanaka and Atsushi Nambu
Division of System Neurophysiology, National Institute for Physiological Sciences and Department of Physiological Sciences, Graduate University for Advanced Studies (SOKENDAI), Okazaki, Japan

* Corresponding Author

Masahiko Inase
Department of Physiology, Kinki University School of Medicine, Osaka-Sayama, Japan

5. References

[1] Alexander GE, DeLong MR, Strick PL. Parallel organization of functionally segregated circuits linking basal ganglia and cortex. Annu Rev Neurosci 1986;9: 357-381.
[2] Alexander GE, Crutcher MD. Functional architecture of basal ganglia circuits: neural substrates of parallel processing. Trends Neurosci 1990;13: 266-271.
[3] Parent A, Hazrati L-N. Functional anatomy of the basal ganglia. I. The cortico-basal ganglia-thalamo-cortical loop. Brain Res Rev 1995;20: 91-127.
[4] Mink JW. The basal ganglia: focused selection and inhibition of competing motor programs. Prog Neurobiol 1996;50: 381-425.
[5] Wise SP. The primate premotor cortex: past, present, and preparatory. Annu Rev Neurosci 1985;8:1-19.
[6] Caminiti R, Ferraina S, Mayer AB. Visuomotor transformations: early cortical mechanisms of reaching. Curr Opin Neurobiol 1998;8:753-761.
[7] Hoshi E, Tanji J. Distinctions between dorsal and ventral premotor areas: anatomical connectivity and functional properties. Curr Opin Neurobiol 2007;17:234-242.
[8] Cisek P, Kalaska JF. Neural mechanisms for interacting with a world full of action choices. Annu Rev Neurosci 2010;33:269-298.
[9] Matelli M, Luppino G, Rizzolatti G. Patterns of cytochrome oxidase activity in the frontal agranular cortex of the macaque monkey. Behav Brain Res 1985;18: 125-136.
[10] Barbas H, Pandya DN. Architecture and frontal cortical connections of the premotor cortex (area 6) in the rhesus monkey. J Comp Neurol 1987;256: 211-228.
[11] Hashimoto M, Takahara D, Hirata Y, Inoue K, Miyachi S, Nambu A, Tanji J, Takada M, Hoshi E. Motor and nonmotor projections from the cerebellum to rostrocaudally distinct sectors of the dorsal premotor cortex in macaques. Eur J Neurosci 2010;31:1402-1413.
[12] Nambu A, Takada M, Inase M, Tokuno H. Dual somatotopical representations in the primate subthalamic nucleus: evidence for ordered but reversed body-map transformations from the primary motor cortex and the supplementary motor area. J Neurosci 1996;16:2671-2683.
[13] Nambu A, Tokuno H, Inase M, Takada M. Corticosubthalamic input zones from forelimb representations of the dorsal and ventral divisions of the premotor cortex in the macaque monkey: comparison with the input zones from the primary motor cortex and the supplementary motor area. Neurosci Lett 1997;239: 13-16.
[14] Takada M, Tokuno H, Nambu A, Inase M. Corticostriatal projections from the somatic motor areas of the frontal cortex in the macaque monkey: segregation versus overlap of

input zones from the primary motor cortex, the supplementary motor area, and the premotor cortex. Exp Brain Res 1998;120: 114-128.

[15] Takada M, Tokuno H, Nambu A, Inase M. Corticostriatal input zones from the supplementary motor area overlap those from the contra- rather than ipsilateral primary motor cortex. Brain Res 1998;791: 335-340.

[16] Takada M, Tokuno H, Hamada I, Inase M, Ito Y, Imanishi M, Hasegawa N, Akazawa T, Hatanaka N, Nambu A. Organization of inputs from cingulate motor areas to basal ganglia in macaque monkey. Eur J Neurosci 2001;14:1633-1650.

[17] Inase M, Tokuno H, Nambu A, Akazawa T, Takada M. Corticostriatal and corticosubthalamic input zones from the presupplementary motor area in the macaque monkey: comparison with the input zones from the supplementary motor area. Brain Res 1999;833: 191-201.

[18] Tachibana Y, Nambu A, Hatanaka N, Miyachi S, Takada M. Input–output organization of the rostral part of the dorsal premotor cortex, with special reference to its corticostriatal projection. Neurosci Res 2004;48: 45-57.

[19] Saga Y, Hirata Y, Takahara D, Inoue K, Miyachi S, Nambu A, Tanji J, Takada M, Hoshi E. Origins of multisynaptic projections from the basal ganglia to rostrocaudally distinct sectors of the dorsal premotor area in macaques. Eur J Neurosci 2011;33: 285-297.

[20] Hoshi E, Tanji J. Differential involvement of neurons in the dorsal and ventral premotor cortex during processing of visual signals for action planning. J Neurophysiol 2006;95: 3596-3616.

[21] Matelli M, Govoni P, Galletti C, Kutz DF, Luppino G. Superior area 6 afferents from the superior parietal lobule in the macaque monkey. J Comp Neurol 1998;402: 327-352.

[22] Luppino G, Rozzi S, Calzavara R, Matelli M. Prefrontal and agranular cingulate projections to the dorsal premotor areas F2 and F7 in the macaque monkey. Eur J Neurosci 2003;17: 559-578.

[23] Kaneda K, Nambu A, Tokuno H, Takada M. Differential processing patterns of motor information via striatopallidal and striatonigral projections. J Neurophysiol 2002;88: 1420-1432.

[24] Yelnik J, Percheron G, Francois C. A Golgi analysis of the primate globus pallidus. II. Quantitative morphology and spatial orientation of dendritic arborizations. J Comp Neurol 1984;227: 200-213.

[25] Yelnik J, Francois C, Percheron G, Heyner S. Golgi study of the primate substantia nigra. I. Quantitative morphology and typology of nigral neurons. J Comp Neurol 1987;265:455-472.

[26] Hazrati L-N, Parent A. Convergence of subthalamic and striatal efferents at pallidal level in primates: an anterograde double-labeling study with biocytin and PHA-L. Brain Res 1992;569: 336-340.

[27] Bolam JP, Hanley JJ, Booth PA, Bevan MD. Synaptic organisation of the basal ganglia. J Anat 2000;196 (Pt 4): 527-542.

[28] Parent A, Sato F, Wu Y, Gauthier J, Levesque M, Parent M. Organization of the basal ganglia: the importance of axonal collateralization. Trends Neurosci 2000;23: S20-27.